The Myth of Osteoporosis

What every woman needs to know about creating bone health

THE MYTH OF OSTEOPOROSIS

No part of this book is intended to be a substitute for medical advice, diagnosis, or treatment. Every individual is unique, and no book can possibly address each person's special situation. Do not make changes in your medications or lifestyle without consulting your health care provider. The information contained in this book is intended to stimulate discussion with your health care providers, and not to replace their advice.

Copyright © 2022

All rights reserved. No part of this book may be reproduced or utilized in any form or by any means, electronic or mechanical, including photocopying, recording, or by any information storage or retrieval system, without permission in writing from the Publisher.

Table of Contents
Section I: Major Myths

CHAPTER 1: A Family Story
CHAPTER 2: The Myth of Risk
CHAPTER 3: The Myth of Diagnosis
CHAPTER 4: The Myth of Causality

Section II: Treatment Myths

CHAPTER 5: Overview of Drug Treatments
CHAPTER 6: The Myth of Safety
CHAPTER 7: The Myth of the Magic Bullet

Section III: Creating Bone Health

CHAPTER 8: Understanding Health
CHAPTER 9: Positive Reactions
CHAPTER 10: Creating Strong Bones
CHAPTER 11: A Family Story, 10 Years Later

***

Section I: Major Myths

Chapter 1
A Family Story

It was 1994, and I was relaxing at home with friends, when my 16-year-old daughter rang from the Auckland Hospital fracture clinic. She had been having a follow-up visit for a wrist fracture sustained on the ski slopes a few weeks previously – her sixth fracture. It was the normal sort of teenage call: "I won't be home for a while," she said, "I am going into town to meet some friends." She added: "Oh, and by the way, the doctor who looked at my X-ray says that I have the bones of an 80 year old."

I was speechless, devastated, and immediately stricken with guilt. I assumed my daughter's condition was due to bad mothering. I immediately started examining how I had raised her. Or was it my diet during pregnancy that was at fault? I had always been conscientious about giving my children good food, but maybe I had made some critical mistake. My fears were irrational of course but had many questions and few answers. I was determined, however, to learn all I could about osteoporosis. That phone call became the impetus for this book.

In the meantime, my daughter became justifiably frightened. She was young, alone, and had no context in which to gauge her diagnosis. Believing her fragile bones could not withstand any knocks or pressure, she immediately cut back on physical activity – contrary to what she ought to have done, yet no such advice was given. (Years later, when I consider this event, I am appalled by the thoughtlessness of how she was told of her condition.)

A bone densitometry scan confirmed that she had very low bone mineral density for her age. Extremely low bone density in young people is a concern because it means they haven't achieved the recognized normal, healthy peak bone mass to take them through to adulthood and older age when bone density naturally declines and fracture risk increases. Initially, we were told that existing bone mass is like a bank account which can be drawn on. In my daughter's case, according to current understanding, she was already in debt.

The family participated in a study at the endocrinology department at Auckland hospital to determine a genetic risk factor. Measuring the bone densities of the entire extended family revealed that my three siblings, parents, husband, son, daughter, and I have varying degrees of low bone mineral density (BMD), culminating most seriously in my son and daughter. Six of us have osteoporosis as defined by a BMD of -2.5 standard deviations (SD) below norm or less, and the rest of us have what is called osteopenia, or low bone density, a BMD of -1 SD to -2.5 SDs.

Growing up, my sister, brother, and I routinely broke wrists, the occasional digit, leg, or collarbone, and accepted that this was normal childhood wear and tear. In our small town of 14,000 inhabitants, we rather proudly held the record for the most X-rays at the local hospital. The fracturing eased off as we became adults, and when my children in turn started occasionally breaking their limbs, I stoically assumed the role of fracture-clinic mother, believing this was all a normal part of parenting.

Identifying idiopathic osteoporosis (osteoporosis of unknown origin) in our family raised many questions but provided no answers. Efforts to determine a cause were inconclusive. Blood DNA samples from individuals in the family and other similarly affected families were sent to Oxford, England, to screen for a common genetic factor. Researchers determined that there was a genetic link – though they were unsuccessful in isolating such a gene.[1]

For my children it was difficult to know what action to take. There wasn't any known treatment for very low bone density in a young person. All the tested, prescribed treatments were for postmenopausal women with low bone density. Hormonal treatments were inappropriate, and it wasn't clear that non-hormonal treatments would be effective in a person her age. I also remained unconvinced that the recommended drug (a bisphosphonate) would be safe, given the current lack of data on its use in young people.

I began to look deeper into possible causes of osteoporosis, ever conscious that the years when peak bone mass is established in a young person (up to about age 20) were almost over for my children. My daughter's situation was identified as more serious than her brother's. His bone mass was low, though hers was significantly lower. Further, a young female can be at risk for additional bone loss during pregnancy, and may lose bone mass more rapidly after menopause.

Primarily, this book is the result of my search to uncover answers for the members of my family who have this diagnosis – relatives such as my oldest sister, now postmenopausal, who had experienced increased loss of bone density in her spine, yet found herself in the difficult position of having to make treatment decisions on the basis of little information.

When I began my research, I quickly learned that members of my family were not the only ones who were worried about their bone health. As a women's health educator I conduct seminars and workshops in the community to help women manage the menopause transition and stay well in the years to follow. The subject of osteoporosis was always raised in my classes, evoking feelings of anxiety and fear among many women who were convinced that, by virtue of their age alone, they were candidates for osteoporosis once they passed through menopause. For most women, the question was not whether they were at risk for osteoporosis, but what to do about the impending condition. I would later discover that the widespread notion that all women are at risk for osteoporosis is a myth – though not the only one.

In discussions those days, hormone replacement therapy (HRT) attracted much attention. For decades, women had taken HRT to relieve symptoms associated with menopause. Increasing numbers of women, however, were also taking HRT to prevent postmenopausal diseases such as heart disease and osteoporosis. Questions arose. Should women take HRT following a diagnosis of low bone density? Would HRT prevent osteoporosis? Was the hormone therapy linked to an increased risk for breast cancer? There seemed to be many information gaps, and women often joked that they felt between a rock and a hard place, that the choices were too difficult.

Then came a revelation. My son was staying in a cabin on a lake in Manitoba, Canada, for a weekend. Among the magazines in the cabin was a Homemakers magazine with a cover article by journalist Elaine Dewar titled "Breaking News – Blowing the Whistle on Osteoporosis." He mailed me the article, which called into question the accuracy of bone density testing diagnoses. The article referred to a large Canadian study that found DXA machines using manufacturer's reference standards for measuring bone density were diagnosing up to three times as many cases of osteoporosis than when an independent Canadian reference standard was used. The findings were significant: osteoporosis had come to be defined by measure of low bone density, though DXA manufacturers had not standardized their machines.

Suddenly I realized that every aspect of the disease was up for debate. Was osteoporosis as prevalent as people were being led to believe? Were people who were not at risk being prescribed medication? Was bone density even an accurate predictor of osteoporosis? If low bone density was not necessarily a cause for concern, why were drugs to increase bone density being prescribed so readily? What did this mean for my parents, my sister, my son and daughter? What did it mean for the millions of women who were being tested and told they had the disease? Why was nobody questioning how osteoporosis had gone from being rare, to being everywhere?

The more I read, the more I was convinced that women and their doctors were misinformed. I uncovered increasing amounts of evidence that well women were being frightened into unnecessary testing, handed questionable diagnoses, and urged to undergo long-term treatments for a disease that they probably didn't have. I discovered that there are many risk factors for osteoporosis in addition to low bone density, and that when osteoporosis is defined as a condition of fragile bones that fracture easily it is, in fact, a rare disease.

One day I had a major breakthrough. I was spending hours each week in the Auckland medical school library searching medical journals, unearthing articles, and following any lead, reference or footnote that would provide further insight into the disease. An article referred to a 1997 report by the British Columbia Office of Health Technology Assessment. The independent, government-funded agency reviewed evidence to determine the effectiveness of bone mineral density testing. The agency reported that BMD testing does not accurately identify women who will go on to fracture as they age – a finding that prompted a CBC documentary that alerted the public to what it called "the marketing of fear" to well women. The report referred to a study that had found that the cracks in Vancouver's sidewalks were more likely to cause hip fractures in the elderly than low bone density, and that screening large populations of menopausal women for osteoporosis might only prevent between 1 percent and 5 percent of fractures in the elderly. The review raised concerns about over-diagnosis of the disease and over-prescribing of medication and addressed the issue of the ineffectiveness of current drug therapies. Similar reviews in countries including the United States, United Kingdom, France, Sweden, and Australia reached the same conclusions - though the results of these government-funded projects rarely rated a mention in the press. The overriding message remained that BMD testing was a reliable and effective way to diagnosis osteoporosis.

My attention moved to the popular treatments for osteoporosis – HRT, bisphosphonates, and the much-heralded prevention strategies of calcium and dairy consumption. There was little evidence to recommend the widely advertised pharmaceuticals or the daily taking of calcium. Coming from a dairy-producing nation that readily accepts the claim that milk consumption results in healthy bones, I was particularly stunned to find that the evidence in favor of dairy just wasn't there. My greatest concern however was for the millions of women worldwide who were trustingly taking hormone replacement therapy in the belief that it was protecting their bones. There was minimal evidence that HRT prevented fractures, and there was a growing body of evidence that it caused breast cancer and heart disease.

Then in July 2002 the National Institutes of Health released startling findings from its Women's Health Initiative – one of the largest studies of its kind ever undertaken. Researchers announced that HRT use was linked to an increased risk for breast cancer, heart disease, clotting, and stroke. Doctors' offices and clinics were flooded with calls from worried women who had been taking HRT in the belief that it was keeping them well. Many women stopped HRT and were in great need of information and reassurance.

In the months that followed, I spent many hours talking to women and listening to their stories as part of a national campaign to disseminate accurate information. Some women had been taking HRT for 20 years or more but had no idea why. Others believed HRT to be a wonder drug that would keep them youthful while preventing menopausal discomfort and age-related diseases. Many women felt depressed, fearful and betrayed. Now, many women had to decide which treatment, if any, to undertake. Osteoporosis-preventing drugs such as the bisphosphonates Fosamax, Actonel and Boniva quickly filled the void left by HRT. But how safe and effective were they? Was it a case of out of the frying pan and into the fire?

Eight years down the track as I update this book I find that little has changed. Osteoporosis is still a controversial condition, trumpeted by drug companies, frontline advocacy groups and clinicians as a silent but deadly disease that stands to destroy the lives of tens of millions of postmenopausal women. The osteoporosis market continues to expand to include those with osteopenia or low bone density. Untold numbers of fearful individuals now take osteoporosis drugs, while massive profits continue to roll in for the drug companies. Annual sales of these drugs reached a staggering US$8.3 billion in 2009.

Yet the majority of those millions of people taking bisphonates and other drug treatments will not benefit. For the few fractures that may be prevented in a small percentage of people, many more fractures still occur. No drug prevents falls, and there is still no drug on the market that will prevent hip fractures. Meanwhile a lengthening litany of risks associated with bisphosphonates: chronic and acute joint bone and muscle pain, sudden fractures of the femur, atrial fibrillation, rare but catastrophic osteonecrosis of the jaw, inflammatory eye disease, and cancer of the esophagus have the very experts who previously strenuously promoted them now suggesting users consider a 'drug holiday' after 5 years. They also suggest new drugs in the wings as alternatives. Drugs like Prolia (or denosumab), a newly FDA approved genetically engineered human monoclonal antibody that profoundly suppresses bone remodelling. It comes onto the market with no long-term testing, but an FDA review cautions that is likely to cause osteonecrosis of the jaw, spontaneous atypical fractures, and delayed healing as bisphosphonates have. In addition there is a risk of infections and cancers.

Bone mineral density (BMD) testing is as blunt a tool as ever. Large studies reveal that the vast majority of fractures occur in those with normal, slightly low, or even high bone density. BMD testing has been widely discredited as an accurate means to determine who will go on to fracture, but it remains the standard diagnostic tool. Additional multi-factorial questionnaire-type tools like the World Health Organization's fracture risk algorithm (FRAX) use web technology, i-Phone and i-Pad apps to reach the masses. But FRAX is proving controversial as well. Criteria take into account factors such as being white, female, smoking and drinking habits, weight, personal fracture history, and whether parents ever fractured (with no distinction between high or low trauma fracture). There are concerns that the criteria are insufficient, that the formula on which the tool is based is faulty, and that the advised threshold for medication in the US is far too low, allowing for people who are not at risk of osteoporosis to be identified as candidates for treatment. The U.S. Preventive Services Task Force recommendations for osteoporosis screening in 2011 have been greatly expanded, risking turning millions of healthy women into patients. They now include all women over age 65, and women over the age of 50 identified as having some risk factors.

There is some good news. Hip fracture incidence in the US has continued to decline over the past 20 years. It is not clear why, but widespread efforts to prevent the elderly from falling including exercise programs, safer environments, better nutrition, and addressing the issues of polypharmacy in the elderly may be paying off. There is also good evidence that adequate levels of vitamin D may reduce falls and hip fractures, at least in part by reversing muscle weakness. Generally there is much greater awareness of the importance of good bone nutrition including a range of essential nutrients, not just calcium. And an understanding of the secondary causes of osteoporosis is leading many to eliminate these factors before embarking on treatment of low bone density alone.

Osteoporosis is not a killer disease. Bones break. They are designed to do so when struck in a particular way. And bones heal. Although painful at the time, fractures heal remarkably well in most cases, and even osteoporotic bone will repair itself. Young people and old people break bones. Genuine vertebral fractures can be very painful, but with rest and time they heal. These days most hip fractures are skilfully repaired with routine hip replacement procedures. I have watched my 88 year-old mother and my mother-in-law both sustain hip fractures then walk a few steps the day after surgery (with assistance). I have seen whole wards of elderly women up and walking within days of their fracture. When a person is generally well prior to fracturing, they can expect to make a good recovery. (My mother returned to driving her car six weeks after her hip fracture.) When there are multiple issues contributing to the frailty of a person then a hip fracture can be the proverbial last straw. But just how the National Osteoporosis Foundation justifies its frightening website slogan "24 percent of hip fracture patients age 50 and over die in the year following their fracture" is a mystery.

Claims of an epidemic of osteoporosis are believed by many to be 'disease-mongering'. People are constantly breaking bones as a result of accidents and falls. Determining whether a fracture is a result of low or high impact is an issue that gets little attention so it isn't hard to present high rates of fracture. In the last 20 years a single risk factor (low bone density) has been transformed into a medical disease in order to sell tests and drugs to well women. It has been easy to frighten an entire population of ageing women into believing they are at risk of a deadly disease.

I have written this book to provide accurate, important information. I encourage women to learn the facts about osteoporosis so that they can see through many of the myths surrounding the disease. I encourage women and men to question a diagnosis of osteoporosis and of osteopenia. Most importantly, I encourage everyone to investigate all options for staying well and maintaining excellent bone health.

***

Chapter 2
The Myth of Risk

Myth #1: Every woman over the age of 50 is at risk for osteoporosis.

At age 45, Ann agreed to have a bone density scan. Her doctor recommended it and emphasized that it was the responsible thing for women her age to do as they approach menopause. As Ann pulled herself off the radiology table after her bone densitometry test, the technician assessing the computerized results warned her that by the time she was 80 she could "be in big trouble." Ann felt shocked and anxious. A follow-up visit to a specialist confirmed that she had "decreased bone density" and included advice that she should immediately begin a calcium supplement program and return for a scan in two years to monitor a potentially serious situation. Her low bone density was blamed on a lifelong aversion to dairy products and two back-to-back pregnancies, followed by lengthy periods of breastfeeding.

Ann is a very fit person with a small build and no family history of osteoporosis. She lacks risk factors for the disease — she doesn't smoke, drink, or take any medications, and she has an excellent diet. She has had no personal history of low-trauma fractures, a sign associated with the disease. Ann does not have osteoporosis. She has osteopenia, or low bone density, and even that diagnosis is questionable given the wide variation of measurements with bone densitometry (DXA) machines [1]. Furthermore, this level of bone density may be normal for her. Importantly, the test did not tell her about the strength of her bones — DXA is not able to do that.

There is something deeply disturbing about being told that you have osteoporosis, particularly in the absence of symptoms or disease. It is like hearing that your cherished family home is structurally unsound, that termites have eaten away at the foundation and it could collapse at any time. With your house, you can always move to another building, but when it comes to your body, moving out is not an option.

The effect of a diagnosis of osteoporosis can be shattering but little attention has been paid to the psychological impact of such a diagnosis. One study showed that many women stopped exercising, avoided lifting heavy objects, and generally limited physical activity after being told they were at risk for fracture — the very opposite of what is recommended [2]. Others immediately embark upon long-term drug regimens that may carry risks far more serious than a broken wrist bone or a loss of height [3].

What the specialist could have done was reassure Ann that her bones are probably normal for a small-framed person [4]. He could have told her that bone mineral density (BMD) is only a small part of the osteoporosis story. Lacking other risk factors, her chances of fracturing because of fragile bones were minimal [5]. Had he advised her according to the evidence, he would have told her there is no evidence that dairy foods reduce the risk of fracture [6]. In fact, he would have acknowledged that her diet was more than adequate. He could have reassured her that, even though bone density may be lost during pregnancy and lactation, it recovers quickly, regardless of the interval between pregnancies [7]. He could have encouraged her to remain fit and to do weight-bearing exercise. If she wanted to take anything, he could have recommended. a balanced bone nutrient supplement. Instead, he has added her to the ever-growing list of "worried well" women who believe themselves candidates for a crippling disease.

Fifty years ago osteoporosis was rare. Doctors considered it an uncommon bone disease, not a women's disease. Until 25 years ago, most of us had never heard of it. Spontaneous fracturing of hips or compressing of vertebrae resulting in painful curvature of the spine was unusual and confined to the very elderly. In contrast, osteoporosis foundations throughout the world now warn of an epidemic. Frightening slogans on the National Osteoporosis Foundation website in 2011 assert that one in two women (and one in four men) will suffer an osteoporosis related fracture in their lifetime, and that "24 percent of hip fracture patients over age 50 will die within the year following their fracture" [8]. Statistics like these suggest that the disease is more widespread and more devastating than breast cancer, AIDS, and heart disease combined. How did this happen? More importantly, is it true? If so, surely our hospital beds should be full of people with fractures, and most elderly women should have severely curved spines (dowager's humps).

Frontline osteoporosis organizations predict that there will be a 50 percent increase in the disease in the next 15 years. World elderly populations are growing, consistent with the global population explosion of the last 50 years. It is estimated that 1.7 million hip fractures were suffered by senior citizens in the world in 1990. That number is expected to increase to 6 million by 2050 *based solely on increasing populations and increased life expectancy* [9]. The expanded populations in Asia, Africa, and South America are predicted to lead to massive increases in the numbers of elderly people. Consequently, there is an expected shifting of the "burden of the osteoporosis disease" from the developed world to the developing world, despite the very low rates of fracture in these countries. The incidence of hip fracture in Mainland China remains one of the lowest in the world [10]. Yet the International Osteoporosis Foundation projects that more than about 50 percent of all osteoporotic hip fractures will occur in Asia by the year 2050[11].

Yet hip fracture rates are actually falling in North America! In good news that rarely makes the headlines, hip fracture rates have fallen by 32 percent in women and by 25 percent in men over two decades in Canada (since 1985) and a similar trend has been observed in the United States [12].

Osteoporosis

While osteoporosis has been present in human populations for thousands of years, it has always been recorded as affecting only a small fraction of the population. Although there is little recorded evidence of the disease in antiquity, in a rare find, the skeleton of a postmenopausal woman from Lisht, Upper Egypt, dated to the 12th Dynasty (1990–1786 B.C.), has been scanned to reveal a hip fracture and compression fractures of some of the vertebrae [13].

Osteoporosis used to be defined as a *disease* where bones fracture as a result of little impact because they have become thin, brittle, and have lost tensile strength. Today's definition of osteoporosis defines it as a *condition* characterized by low bone density or reduced bone quantity. This definition says nothing about bone quality — that is, its strength or brittleness. It also says very little about the likelihood of fracture,

Everybody loses bone density as they age, but the vast majority of the population don't fracture as a result of low bone density. When characterized as a condition of fragile bones, the disease osteoporosis is uncommon in women under the age of 80. After age 80, most fractures are likely to occur due to factors that predispose someone to falling, such as poor eyesight, dementia, and medications like sleeping pills and antidepressants. Other factors associated with frailty such as immobility and malnutrition can further contribute to thinning of bone, as can medications such as corticosteroids. Under these conditions, almost any elderly person may fall and fracture his or her hip. The older and more unwell a person is, the greater the risk of fracture. Maintaining a good level of health and fitness will help a well person in their 50s and 60s avert such an event.

Osteoporosis is thought of as a disease when in most cases, it is just a condition. People are diagnosed with osteoporosis because they have low bone density, not because they have fractured. This occurs routinely despite the fact that

BMD testing does not accurately identify women who will go on to fracture [14].

A person with high bone density may fracture, and another with low bone density may never fracture. Low BMD is but one of many risk factors for a disease that can only be truly diagnosed when there is a "fragility" fracture — a fracture resulting from low impact or trauma. Calling a measure of low BMD osteoporosis is like calling elevated cholesterol heart disease, or high blood pressure a stroke.

When it is characterized by fragile bones that break easily, osteoporosis is a serious disease with potentially devastating consequences. But since osteoporosis was redefined as normal age-related bone loss, the worried well now have a new diagnosis. A vast number of supposedly at-risk people are encouraged to take expensive tests and drugs to prevent something that most of them will probably never have.

The vast majority of postmenopausal women need not be concerned about osteoporosis. There is substantial evidence that a good diet, healthy lifestyle, and regular exercise are sufficient protection against future fracture. Many experts agree. Mark Helfand, one of the members of the U.S. National Institutes of Health (NIH) consensus panel on the prevention, diagnosis and treatment of osteoporosis, stated in a Washington Post article: "I think even people who agree that osteoporosis is a serious health problem can still say it is being hyped. It is hyped. Most of what you could do to prevent osteoporosis later in life has nothing to do with getting a test or taking a drug [15]."

Misleading Information

The information from the osteoporosis literature, most doctors, advertising, and the media is misleading and most often inaccurate. These inaccuracies have been allowed to proliferate unchecked without public policy intervention or objective analysis. Challenging evidence has been published repeatedly in prestigious medical journals. Still, the message that predominates is the myth that virtually all women more than 50 years old face the specter of debilitating pain, loss of independence, and immobility. Evidence-based articles contradict many commonly held beliefs about the prevalence, diagnosis, and treatment of osteoporosis. This other side of the story is known to the best osteoporosis specialists and those who stay informed. It has been published in the medical literature, discussed at conferences, yet has somehow failed to filter through to the public. Most ill-informed appear to be the doctors who help "at-risk" patients make decisions regarding their bone health. Too often they base decisions on misinformation, not facts.

A massive osteoporosis-preventing industry has emerged based on the myth of risk. This industry can only increase in size, as more and more of the graying female baby boom population acquire the low bone density "risk factor" for osteoporosis — simply by virtue of their age. Consequently, age is seen as reason enough to perpetuate the idea that hip fracture and subsequent disability are inevitable, unless steps are taken to avoid them.

Promulgating the Myth

In the early 1980s, most women had never heard of osteoporosis, and doctors saw very few patients with the disease. But that was about to change. In 1982, a major promotional campaign sponsored by pharmaceutical companies producing hormone replacement therapy (HRT) set out to create public awareness of osteoporosis as an important women's health issue. The campaign included massive radio, television, and magazine coverage with articles and advertisements published in Vogue, McCall's, and Reader's Digest. Although the campaign focused on the disfigurement of the dowager's hump and the damage of the disease, the companies clearly stood to benefit from increasing public awareness of this condition. Fearful women who went to their doctors to discuss prevention were likely to end up with a prescription for

HRT. Yet astoundingly, there was no evidence from placebo-controlled trials that hormone replacement would even prevent or treat osteoporosis.

So successful was the campaign that by the mid-1980s most European and American women had not only heard of the disease, they were increasingly fearful of it. They were convinced of the apparent inevitability of hip fractures and were frightened of becoming like the elderly woman with the severely bent spine seen in calcium advertisements. The medical profession in turn was convinced that osteoporosis was reaching epidemic proportions and their role was to identify and treat these patients.

In their review of the evidence for the effectiveness of bone mineral density testing, the British Columbia Office of Health Technology Assessment quotes from a report:

Many advertisements play on the fear of aging, such as the spot for a calcium supplement that shows a healthy 30-year-old women transformed to a stooped 65-

year-old in 30 seconds. While such an image capitalizes on the fear of losing youthful beauty, it draws on even deeper fears of disability leading to loss of independence.

The information on hip fractures is equally frightening. For example, a popular guide to preventing osteoporosis states: "The consequences of osteoporosis can be devastating. Fewer than one-half of all women who suffer a hip fracture regain normal function. Fifteen percent die shortly after their injury, and nearly 30 percent die within a year." The fear for women is that even if they survive a hip fracture, they may face long years of dependency and immobility [16].

The advertisements fail to mention that the majority of postmenopausal women who do have spinal (vertebral) fractures are unaware of the fact and have no symptoms. They also ignore the fact that most fractures occur only in the very elderly and are linked to many other complicating factors. The truth is that most women who suffer hip fractures are aged

80 or older and are unwell. Many of the women who did not recover had been in declining health preceding their fractures. While a hip fracture was part of the disability surrounding their deaths, it did not cause them. It is estimated that as few as 14 percent of deaths following a hip or pelvic fracture occur in women who are healthy prior to the event [17].

Advertisements, media campaigns, and fact sheets in doctors' waiting rooms grossly exaggerate the numbers of people who fracture and the impact that osteoporosis can have on a postmenopausal woman's life.

The Redefining of Osteoporosis

Normal: A value for bone mineral density or content within 1 standard deviation (SD) of the young adult reference mean.

Osteopenia: A value for bone mineral density or content more than 1 SD below the young adult mean but less than 2.5 SD below this value.

Osteoporosis: A value for bone mineral density or content 2.5 SD or more below the young adult mean.

Severe (Established) Osteoporosis: A value for bone mineral density or content 2.5 SD or more below the young adult mean in the presence of one or more fragility fractures.

In 1994, in the wake of the globally successful osteoporosis marketing campaign, a new definition of osteoporosis was created that was so broad that it would diagnose half of all postmenopausal women as diseased. Osteoporosis had previously been characterized by fragility fractures — that is, bones breaking under relatively low impact. Examples of fragility fractures include falling off a chair, tripping while walking, or stubbing your toe with resultant fracture. In contrast, high-impact trauma is when you fracture your leg in a skiing accident, or your ribs in a car accident. High-impact trauma represents conditions under which any bone would break.

In 1988, Dual X-ray Absorptiometry (DXA) machinery was developed to measure the bone mineral density (BMD) of an individual to determine the likelihood that a person will develop osteoporosis. DXA has become the internationally recognized gold standard for determining osteoporosis risk. But BMD only measures bone mass, not the factors which contribute to bone fragility, such as bone size and shape, vertebral body diameter, hip axis length and loss of trabecular cross-bracing.

Bone mineral density naturally decreases with age in most people, but not all people are at risk for fragility fractures. The impressive development of sophisticated DXA technology had created the potential for measuring low BMD. This allowed low bone mineral density to take a quantum leap from the category of a hidden risk factor to the category of an easily diagnosed disease.

In 1994, a World Health Organization (WHO) committee of experts established an international standard that now gives a bone mineral density reading 2.5 standard deviations below "normal" a diagnosis of *osteoporosis*. Readings 1.0 to 2.5 standard deviations below normal are classified as *osteopenia*, or low bone density — the early stage of osteoporosis. An assumed average peak bone density of young white women currently determines the normal level. This is known as a T-score. For each standard deviation decrease in bone mineral density, doctors are warned that fracture risk in their patient is predicted to double [18]. This means that unless women maintain their bone mass at peak levels throughout their life span, they will be labeled at risk or diseased. The natural biological variation among healthy adults and the normal age-related bone loss are not accounted for by this definition. Neither is the all-important fact that low bone density is not a good predictor of future fracture.

The new definition meant that millions of women suddenly qualified for diagnosis of a disease for which they had never considered themselves at risk. As one osteoporosis authority put it: "If you want to make more people have osteoporosis, simply change the definition of osteoporosis or use a kind of bone density measurement that decreases with age [i.e., the T-Score] [19]."

Both these things have happened. The definition of osteoporosis has changed from fragility fractures to a measure of bone density. The "normal" level is a young Causasian person with high bone density. That ensures that age-related decrease in bone density is automatically categorized as abnormal.

The impact of redefining osteoporosis was considerable. Once a woman is diagnosed as having low bone density, she is likely to be hooked into a lifetime of screening, monitoring, and drug therapy. Based in large part on the redefinition, some 37 percent (16 million) of all U.S. postmenopausal women were taking hormone replacement therapy (HRT) to prevent osteoporosis by 1999, and by 2000, HRT had become the No. 1 prescription drug in the world [20] [21]. Since 2002 prescriptions have dropped by about half, but the number of U.S. women on HRT remained at almost 10 million in 2009, despite the Women's Health Initiative Study having demonstrated that long-term use of HRT is not safe [22] [23]. New drugs have taken the place of HRT and from 2003 to 2009 annual sales of osteoporosis drugs have about doubled with worldwide sales reaching $8.3 billion [24].

One assumes that the World Health Organization is an independent and neutral body, untainted by any conflict of interest in its assessments and reports. But the WHO study group on bone densitometry screening that defined the thresholds for diagnosing osteoporosis was funded by three major drug companies [25]. From this initial meeting emerged similarly funded conferences worldwide. Despite widespread criticism, this new definition was adopted as the mainstream measure for diagnosing osteoporosis.

At the time many argued against the use of the WHO definition. The Swedish Council on Technology Assessment in Health Care demonstrated that the WHO's use of healthy young women as a reference group resulted in large numbers of women being wrongly defined as abnormal. Using the WHO standards, they estimated that 22 percent of all women over the age of 50 would be defined as having osteoporosis, and 52 percent as having osteopenia. The Swedish council also raised concerns that "defining a complex, often lifelong, process such as osteoporosis in terms of a single BMD measurement is highly problematic and should be critically examined [26]."

The flaws in such a simple definition were many:

1. It assumed that bone density predicts a person's future risk of fracture. We now know it is unable to do that. [27]

2. It assumed that the young reference peak bone mass used in the DXA machine assessment is an accurate representation of everyone's peak bone mass (gained in early adulthood). Peak bone mass, though, is virtually indefinable, as it varies from race to race, between genders, across geographical regions of a country, and even between seasons. Alan Tenenhouse, the principal investigator of a groundbreaking Canadian study: "the most interesting thing we've learned is that peak bone mass varies across the

country... We can't find any real differences to explain it. It's substantial. The difference is greater than 10 percent, which is more than one DXA standard deviation [28]."

3. Astonishingly, there is no international normal reference standard for DXA machines. Manufacturers set their own, often-high standards, resulting in widely varying diagnoses. Results vary between machines, regions, and countries.

4. Most DXA criteria only apply to Caucasian women even though it is known that a huge variation in bone mass exists between ethnic groups. A study of four ethnic groups —Hawaiian, Filipino, Japanese, and Caucasian women — found differences in peak bone mass varying up to 100 percent [29]. It is essential, therefore, that a reference standard based on a local population of the same ethnicity be used when measuring bone density — something that is not commonly done.

The WHO definition was entirely arbitrary. It was apparently never intended to be used for clinical diagnosis but was designed to convince policymakers of the perceived magnitude of the osteoporosis problem. It has since netted far more of the population than was ever anticipated [30]. Despite the anomalies, the osteoporosis societies of the United States and other Western countries relentlessly warned that half of all women over the age of 50 will develop osteoporosis.

In 2008 the WHO created the Fracture Risk Assessment Tool (FRAX) which takes into account ten fracture risk factors in addition to bone density to further assist clinicians to identify those who need treatment. But the 1994 BMD definition remains the mainstream diagnostic tool. Despite its serious limitations, the NOF website in 2011 still declares " A bone density test is the only test that can diagnose osteoporosis before a broken bone occurs [31]."

What About Fracture Rates?

All this is ignoring one essential factor — the presence of low trauma fracture. Because the real concern is breaking bones, the preoccupation with measuring bone mineral density tends to eclipse this obvious and important indicator. You may have low bone density and never fracture; or you may have normal bone density and fracture. Although it is repeatedly overlooked in the publicized WHO definition of osteoporosis, "established osteoporosis" is defined by low BMD *along with one or more fractures resulting from low impact or trauma.*

When determining the incidence of osteoporosis, low bone density is not being distinguished from established osteoporosis, which is defined by the prevalence of fractures. This creates enormous confusion when trying to make sense of osteoporosis statistics, because in most cases, they are based on BMD alone, not fracture rates.

The bone mineral density definition of osteoporosis has contributed to the medicalization of aging women, based on a technology that science has yet to prove is effective. The British Columbia Office of Health Technology Assessment review of the evidence for the effectiveness of bone mineral density testing concludes: "BMD testing is unable to accurately distinguish women at low risk of fracture from those at high risk [32]."

A Caucasian woman's estimated likelihood of an osteoporosis-related fracture after age 50 will depend on the country of residence, the information source, the disease definition, and the interpretation of fracture data. It will range from 10 percent to 56 percent. Most estimates are in the 50 percent range, but fail to explain that this is based on:

* Wrist (or Colles') fractures which tend to happen to women in their 60s and 70s, and may or may not be linked to osteoporosis. There is little evidence that BMD plays a part in these fractures, as DXA measurement of the forearm does not seem to be able to predict them. A Colles' fracture can occur with normal, high, or low bone density of the forearm [33].

*A loose and hotly debated definition of vertebral "fractures." Most vertebral fractures result in loss of height without any major symptoms. No comparison can be made between the seriousness of hip fractures versus vertebral fractures.

According to Dr. Bruce Ettinger, Senior Investigator, Division of Research, Kaiser Permanente Medical Care Program, California, "Only 5 percent to 7 percent of 70-year-olds will show vertebral collapse; only half of these will have two involved vertebrae; and perhaps one-fifth or one-sixth will have symptoms. I have a very big practice and I have very few bent-over patients. There's been a tremendous hullabaloo lately, and there are a lot of worried women — and excessive testing and administration of medications [34]."

* Hip fractures that occur between the age of 80 and 90 are invariably linked to multiple factors. Many elderly people suffer from poor eyesight and other serious medical problems like dementia. Many in this age group are on several prescription medications that can trigger falls and fractures, including corticosteroids, powerful long-acting tranquilizers, and antipsychotics. Falling and breaking a hip, therefore, is most often a marker of generally frail health. In most cases, it has little to do with osteoporosis [35]. In fact, falling in a particular way will fracture the neck of the femur, regardless of bone strength or density.

* A 50-year-old woman has only a 15 percent chance of a hip fracture by the time she is 80. Only a small percentage of that 15 percent will have life-threatening complications from the fracture.

When these factors are taken into account, it is clear that the risk of an osteoporosis-related fracture is nothing near 50 percent. Dr. Bruce Ettinger reassures further: "Women shouldn't worry about osteoporosis. The osteoporosis that causes pain and disability is a very rare disease [36]." Despite this, the media and doctors continue to warn middle-aged women that they must act now to avert a life-threatening disease that can bring death, disability, deformity, and loss of independence.

The absence of internationally agreed criteria for measuring fracture statistics and the debate surrounding the redefinition of osteoporosis as a condition of low bone density has led to widely diverging statistics concerning osteoporosis and osteoporosis-related fractures:

* **The Mayo Clinic:** In the United States, about 21 percent of postmenopausal women have osteoporosis and about 16 per-cent have had a fracture [37].

* **U.S. National Osteoporosis Foundation:** One in two women and one in eight men over age 50 will have an osteoporosis-related fracture in their lifetime [38].

* **The Canadian Multi-Centered Osteoporosis Study:** In Canada, approximately 16 percent of women and 5 percent of men suffer from osteoporosis [39].

***National Health and Nutrition Examination Survey III:** The percentage of adults age 50 years and over with osteoporosis by femur neck BMD are: Men 2 percent (0.8 million adults); Women 10 percent (4.5 million adults) [40].

* **International Osteoporosis Foundation:** Worldwide, the life-time risk for a woman to have an osteoporotic fracture is 30 percent to 40 percent. In men, the risk is about 13 percent [41].

* **National Osteoporosis Society UK:** One in two women and one in five men over the age of 50 in the UK will fracture a bone, mainly as a result of osteoporosis [42].

* **Australian Osteoporosis Society:** It is estimated that the proportion of women with osteoporosis increases from 15 percent in those aged 60 to 64 years up to 71 percent in those more than 80 years of age. The incidence is much lower in men, ranging from 1.6 percent of those aged 60 to 64 years to 19 percent of those aged more than 80 years [43].

* **Osteoporosis New Zealand:** Osteoporosis is a major health issue with 56 percent of all postmenopausal women predicted to have an osteoporosis-related fracture [44].

* **Osteoporosis authority Professor Ian Reid, New Zealand:** "People might be surprised to know that everyone has

osteoporosis, though most to a lesser extent. No one is immune to it really. It is a condition we all have after 40 [45]."

Statements on the incidence of fracture are constructed from data that is open to wide interpretation. Dr. Susan Ott, Associate Professor of Medicine, University of Washington, an international osteoporosis authority, comments:

Counting the actual number of fractures related to osteoporosis is more difficult than it appears and requires strict criteria. It would be quite easy to make the figures high if you wanted. Obviously, a huge number of people fracture as the result of accidents, and who says how many of those should be counted? What actually constitutes a fracture of spinal vertebrae is also dependent upon how the vertebrae are measured. Loss of height has been used as a measure and when a small amount of height loss is applied then fracture rates are very high. However, when stricter criteria involving spinal X-rays and measurement of vertebrae are involved there are far fewer fractures [46].

How do you decide? Dr. R. P. Heaney, osteoporosis expert, writes:

Any bone will break if pressure is applied in a particular way, so falling patterns are also a big factor. Even young normal bone will fracture if struck just so; many elderly fragility fractures are of precisely this sort [47].

Times Have Changed

It is simply not possible to assume that women currently turning 50 will have the same rate of fracture as women who are in the high-risk elderly age group. Those women who are aged 75 to 100 now were born between 1910 and 1935. Their peak bone mass was being developed during a period which spanned the Great Depression and two world wars with the associated poverty, compromised nutrition, and disrupted lifestyles. Who can say that women currently entering menopause are going to have the same fracture rates as their mothers and grandmothers? Chances are they will be very different. This is particularly so, given dietary and lifestyle changes, and the control the baby boomers have had over reproduction, with fewer pregnancies and greater numbers of menstrual periods. Circulating ovarian hormone levels are very different in the woman who is repeatedly pregnant and lactating, and it is well known that reproductive hormones influence bone metabolism. Whether this influences bone health for the better however, is unknown, as is the effect of long-term exposure to synthetic hormones in the form of the oral contraceptive pill, HRT, and environmental hormone-mimicking chemicals.

Women and Aging

Aging in the West is about losses, not gains, and Western clinical medicine has been very influenced by popular perceptions of women and aging. Younger women of reproductive age are considered the standard for what is normal and healthy, and aging women are often considered in terms of hormone deficiency, a condition that needs to be treated with hormone supplements. Reputed to replace the "missing" hormones, HRT had been heralded as the panacea for the aging woman. It promised to deal with menopause discomfort while simultaneously halting age-related bone loss, and by definition, osteoporosis.

The onset of menopause is equated not just with loss of fertility, but also loss of youth, femininity, sexual desirability, and social status. Ours is not a society that tends to place value on life experience and wisdom — thus older women can experience a sense of social redundancy. They often feel a deep fear of disability and the loss of independence.

Magazine articles and books on menopause tend to emphasize the biological changes that occur and perpetuate the idea that the aging female body is in a state of decline. Biological changes associated with aging are discussed in the language of abnormality and decay. Terms such as "failing ovaries" and "estrogen deficiency" label the aging woman as a diseased woman. So entrenched is the idea that the older woman is somehow diseased, that many women expect their minds and bodies to deteriorate after menopause. In the British Columbia Office of Health Technology Assessment's (BCOHTA) review of the evidence for selective BMD testing in Canada, the authors make this point:

The effects of medicalization on a social group can be far-reaching and subtle. For example, as natural phenomena become labeled as disease, anxiety is heightened. The general public is inundated about the "discovered" disease. Social science research of medicine has repeatedly demonstrated how market forces may capitalize on a climate of risk and reassurance, which then drives the use of health technologies regardless of whether they lead to improved health outcome. This has been shown for ultrasound, electronic fetal monitors, predictive genetic screening, and mammography, among others [48].

There is the psychology that if aging is a disease, then it is a potentially curable one. The physician is expected to offer regular screening to monitor the signs of decline and to prescribe treatment to avert diseases.

An associated BCOHTA article puts bone mineral density testing in its social context:

Once the fear of becoming diseased has been created, women are made to feel personally accountable for managing their risk of disease and future illness, and are encouraged to take appropriate measures to prevent it. ... Individuals taking up this burden of preventing sickness and striving more and more to reach the ideal of normality may struggle in vain. The proliferation of disease categories and labels in medicine and psychiatry results in even more restricted definitions of "normal." This leads to increasing numbers of people being labeled abnormal, sick, or deviant. The area of "normality" is shrinking and the area of "abnormality" or less than perfect health is increasing [49].

Research of other cultures indicates that the menopause-associated decline is a uniquely Western phenomenon. In many cultures, the arrival of menopause signals a new freedom. It is associated with an increased social status where women gain worth and veneration. The cultural expectation to live a long and healthy life can be self-fulfilling. Individuals who integrate that expectation do live longer. In traditional Japanese society, for example, women expect to continue to be well. They become respected elders and fulfill a valued role in their communities. Anthropologists also note that menopause passes by unmarked socially or biologically in some cultures. This is particularly so where frequent pregnancy and lactation is the norm. In these cultures, cessation of menstruation is relatively unremarkable [50].

Osteoporosis and Aging

Many countries have not identified osteoporosis as a disease to be concerned about. Rates of fracture are very low in Africa, South America, and most of Asia. In countries like Cambodia, it is reported to be virtually unheard of [51].

Gradual loss of bone density occurs naturally in all males and females with aging, and at varying rates with different bone sites. Some bones actually gain density with age, and others lose very little mass. Age-related bone density loss does not as a matter of course equate with fragility fractures.

The deeply entrenched idea that osteoporosis is reaching epidemic proportions makes it difficult for anyone to seriously challenge the status quo. Women assume that their doctors are fully informed about the prevalence, diagnosis, and treatment of osteoporosis. Virtually no one questions the appropriateness of widespread DXA screening, or the impact of a diagnosis of low bone density on a well woman. The unsuspecting patient and well-intentioned doctor are unaware in most cases that DXA screening is inaccurate and not a good predictor of fracture risk. They simply do not know that frontline therapies for treating osteoporosis have serious associated risks and limited evidence to support their effectiveness in preventing fracture.

The popular public perception is that modern medicine and technology hold the answers to eliminating health risks. But maybe it is time to reconsider. According to an article in the Journal of the American Medical Association, doctors are the third-leading cause of death in the United States, after cancer and heart disease. Every year, 250,000 deaths result from medication errors, errors in hospitals, unnecessary surgery, and the negative effects of drugs. The author of the article, Barbara Starfield, puts the figures in context: Prescription drugs alone claim 106,000 lives annually in the United States. That is equivalent to three jumbo-jet crashes every two days [52].

Women in Western countries have accepted they are at risk for a disease, purely by virtue of their gender and reproductive status. Yet, the evidence that every aspect of the disease is controversial is found throughout the medical literature. The concept that all women over the age of 50 are at risk for osteoporosis is a myth.

***

Chapter 3
The Myth of Diagnosis

Myth #2: Diagnosis of osteoporosis is accurate, reliable, and meaningful.

Osteoporosis is a complex condition that is still not fully understood. Diagnosis is therefore, not as simple as it may appear. A diagnosis of established osteoporosis can only really be made once there has been a fracture as the result of low impact or low trauma, which is confirmation that bone fragility exists. In the absence of such fractures, osteoporosis is invisible and painless, and there is currently still no way to accurately predict who will fracture.

Bone density measurement is a modern phenomenon. We have no idea what the bone densities of our parents or grandparents were as they grew up, or even what our own were as children. Thus, it is difficult to define what is normal during the stages of a given person's lifetime. Because most studies have only measured changes over short periods, and accurate methods for testing bone mineral density have only recently become available, there remains a large gap in understanding bone formation and maintenance over a person's life span. With the availability of bone scanning technology, we are able to measure the bone density of young people as it increases to peak bone mass in young adulthood. But this raises many questions about current understandings of what is normal. Based on the World Health Organization (WHO) definition of osteoporosis, only 84 percent of young women in America are reaching normal levels of bone density [11].

The 1994 WHO definition that characterizes osteoporosis as a measure of BMD, has been adopted throughout the world because BMD is the easiest of the osteoporosis risk factors to measure. Consequently, decades of research, treatment, and preventative approaches have been focused on BMD. Screening and diagnosing of healthy women based on BMD continues despite the widespread discrediting of its ability to predict fracture.

Now doctors can assume responsibility for monitoring and managing the density of their patients' bones from the first DXA scan until the end of their lives. The availability of DXA technology has allowed physicians to begin to identify variations in bone mineral density among populations and to observe changes in an individual over time. However, these observations are of limited value, if they don't help to prevent fragility fractures and reduce the incidence of established osteoporosis. Doctors have the dilemma of determining whether low bone density puts their patient at risk, and whether they should be treated.

Widening the Net

Times are changing in 2011. After years of aggressive promotion of BMD testing as the incontestable method of diagnosing osteoporosis, its validity has been undermined as evidence from several large trials shows that the majority of fractures occur in people with normal, high, or low bone density (osteopenia), not osteoporosis. The National Osteoporosis Risk Assessment (NORA) study of almost 150,000 postmenopausal Caucasian women found that 82 percent of those who fractured did not have a BMD diagnosis of osteoporosis [2]. The five-year US Study of Osteoporotic Fractures (SOF) of 8,065 women over age 65 found that 54 percent of the 243 hip fractures occurred in women who did not have osteoporosis either [3]. And a study of a German health insurance data basis found that out of 7.8 million people diagnosed with osteoporosis only 4.3 percent experienced a clinically recognized fracture [4].

Although BMD testing remains the standard diagnostic test, these outcomes have brought about the development of new tools to consider multiple risk fractures for osteoporosis. And because the large studies have shown that more fractures occur in the vast subset of women with normal to low bone density, there is increased focus on the controversial condition osteopenia, the category of low bone density arbitrarily created by the World Health Organization (WHO) group that re-defined osteoporosis in 1994. (Whereas the threshold for osteoporosis was set at 2.5 standard deviations below the mean for a healthy young adult woman, osteopenia is identified at 1.0 to 2.5 standard deviations below the mean.) Osteopenia is claimed to affect more than half of all postmenopausal women in the United States.

The very same architects of the original WHO definition have now created the Fracture Assessment Tool (FRAX) that uses a variety of factors believed to increase fracture risk (including BMD). The National Osteoporosis Foundation (NOF) has issued new clinicians guidelines incorporating FRAX and BMD which it claims "is most useful in identifying the subset of patients in the low bone mass [osteopenia] category most likely to benefit from treatment [5]." Yet evidence to date has shown the absolute benefit of drug treatment in the osteopenia group to be almost non-existent. It is estimated up to 270 women in this category would need to be treated with bisphosphonate drugs for three years in order to prevent a single vertebral fracture in one of them [6].

The NOF guidelines based on the FRAX algorithm have drawn wide criticism from within the osteoporosis clinical community, as rather than excluding patients at low risk, they run the risk of casting an even wider net and diagnosing and treating much larger populations than those identified by a BMD diagnosis alone [7].

As well as using bone density in its calculation, FRAX identifies 10 factors believed to increase fracture risk independent of bone mineral density:

- Age
- Sex
- Weight and height
- Previous fractures
- Parental hip fracture history
- Smoking status
- Glucocorticoid use
- Rheumatoid arthritis
- Secondary disorders linked to osteoporosis, such as type 1 diabetes
- Drinking three or more alcoholic beverages per day

Individuals and clinicians can access the FRAX website and calculate their risk for fracture. [8] By 2010 the FRAX website was having about 60,000 hits daily, with total cumulative hits of about 200 million. It is even available as an app from the iPhone and iPad from the iTunes App store [9].

But FRAX is proving almost as controversial as the diagnosis of osteopenia. There are concerns that the formula on which the tool is based is faulty. It does not consider factors including vitamin D deficiencies, amount of physical activity and the use of drugs other than glucocorticoids known to cause fracture. It doesn't take the all-important risk factors for falling into account, and neither does it determine whether fractures are a result of low or high trauma. Secondary causes of osteoporosis are limited to a mere few of many.

Despite the flaws, FRAX has been adopted internationally as an adjunct to BMD testing. Individual countries determine the thresholds where treatment is required. This is leading to massive disparity in recommendations from one country to another. A comparison of the US (NOF) and the UK FRAX-based guidelines found that among healthy community dwelling women of average age 74, the US guidelines would determine that 97 percent would be advised to undergo BMD testing, and that 48 percent should be treated. The UK guidelines however, would require that only 13 percent from the same group should have BMD testing and 21 percent of those receive treatment [10].

In the US there have been complaints that the advised threshold for medication is far too low, allowing for people with normal BMD (a T-scores of -1.0 or higher) to be identified as candidates for treatment. The NOF guidelines recommend medication when the calculated risk for hip fracture in the next 10 years is 3 percent or the combined risk of a broken hip, vertebra, shoulder or wrist is 20 percent. When the criteria from the new NOF guidelines were applied to women participants in the large U.S. Study of Osteoporotic Fractures (SOF) it was calculated that **72 percent of white women aged 65 and older, and 93 percent of women aged 75 and over, would be prescribed osteoporosis drugs** [11].

BMD - Only Part of the Story

The WHO officially describes osteoporosis as "a progressive systemic skeletal disease, characterized by low bone mass and micro-architectural deterioration of bone tissue, with a consequent increase in bone fragility and susceptibility to fracture [13]."

This definition identifies two main risk factors — loss of bone quantity and loss of bone quality. DXA scanning measures only bone quantity (bone density or mass), not bone strength. Bone strength is determined by its micro-architecture: its size, shape, trabecular cross bracing, and ability to repair damage. But, because of difficulties in measuring micro-architecture, that important aspect of bone health has been ignored. Bone density alone has been the focus of research and the defining of osteoporosis.

R.P. Heaney, an international expert on osteoporosis, states:

The current prominence of BMD is due to the fact that it can be accurately measured and to some extent controlled. Indeed, essentially all preventative and therapeutic approaches to osteoporosis focus explicitly on acquiring and maintaining bone mass or on restoring lost mass. However, low bone mass probably accounts for less than half of all osteoporotic fractures. Thus history of fracture after age 40 and maternal history of hip fracture are stronger predictors than BMD and are independent of BMD [14].

Indeed, a BMD measurement reveals no information about bone micro-architecture — a DXA scan or an X-ray cannot measure a person's bone quality or strength. Therefore, a person may be low in bone mass, but have perfectly normal bone structure and strength.

With severe osteoporosis, the meshed, inter-linked trabecular bone can erode, greatly weakening the bone. But a DXA scan is not able to identify this type of damage. Typically, osteoporosis literature includes pictures of the various stages of osteoporosis. It shows, as the disease progresses, the increasingly fragile and space-filled lacy network of disconnected trabecular bone. The picture looks as though the bone would disintegrate with the slightest of knocks. These are not images from a DXA scan. They do not relate to diagnoses of osteopenia and osteoporosis. In reality, these familiar images are usually taken from biopsies or autopsies of older people, not from women with DXA diagnoses of low bone density.

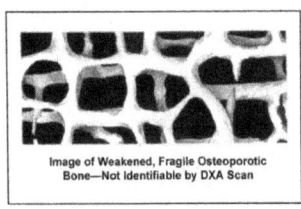

Image of Weakened, Fragile Osteoporotic Bone—Not Identifiable by DXA Scan

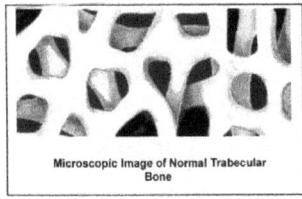

Microscopic Image of Normal Trabecular Bone

Susan Ott, M.D., comments:

Bone quality is determined by bone mass (as measured by bone density) and also by the micro-architecture of bone, the crystal size and shape, the brittleness, the connectivity of the trabecular network, the vitality of the bone cells, ability to repair micro-cracks, and the structure of the bone proteins. The fat cells, vasculature, neuronal pathways, and bone marrow cells probably also influence the quality of the bone as well as the quantity of bone [15].

Range of Normal Bone Mineral Density

Significant and unexplained racial differences exist in both bone mass and the prevalence of fractures. If low bone mass is linked to fracture, then we would expect to see more fractures in ethnic groups that have naturally low bone density. This is not the case. While it is true that people of African descent have higher bone mass and lower rates of fractures, it is also true that Asian women have lower bone mass than Caucasian women, without a proportionally higher rate of hip fractures. Hispanic women have approximately half as many fractures as Caucasian women, but their bone density is no different [16].

In Malmo, Sweden, there is a very high rate of hip fracture — much higher than other Western countries. But a study of the bone mineral density of this population found little evidence that low BMD was the cause. The authors of a study of this phenomenon reported:

The Malmo bone mineral content was on the same level as in the United States, but higher than in Japan and France. The comparatively high level of fragility fractures in the Scandinavian countries cannot be explained by low bone mass [17].

Falling is the big problem with the elderly, not bone density. Because any bone will fracture under certain conditions, a review of 28 studies concluded that most elderly women would fracture with the impact of an unprotected fall. The authors stated:

Differences in bone density between individual women are not great enough to discriminate between who will and who will not later suffer a fracture; this will be determined by chance, by conditions that increase the risk of falling or cause loss of the normal protective reflexes, and by illness and immobility causing bone loss shortly before the fracture [18].

Measuring a man's BMD using DXA scanning is also problematic. Applying the same standard of peak bone mass to the male skeleton, as is done for females, is probably inappropriate. Men generally have taller and larger skeletons than women. Because DXA adjusts for the area scanned, but doesn't completely correct for the fact that wider bones are also thicker, bigger bones appear to have greater BMD, even if the actual tissue density of bone is no different [19].

Furthermore, the more elderly the person, the more difficult it is to accurately measure bone density. Many experts agree that measuring bone mineral density of lumbar spine in the elderly, particularly men, is next to useless. This is because compression fractures, arthritis, and other factors create artificially dense bone in the vertebrae of elderly people.

Bone Densitometry Testing

In 1988, Dual X-ray Absorptiometry (DXA) machinery was developed and quickly became the gold standard to measure bone mineral density (BMD) because of its speed, safety, and perceived accuracy. DXA is sophisticated computerized technology that can, in a matter of minutes and with minimal radiation exposure, measure the mineral content of the vertebrae, the hip, the forearm, or even the whole skeleton. It prints out an impressive computer graphic of the bones and reports where a patient's bone mass falls in relation to the "normal" population. DXA measures the bone mineral content (BMC), then divides that by the surface area of the bone being measured to create a bone mineral density (BMD) measurement expressed in terms of grams per square centimeter. This has limitations, as it provides only a two-dimensional reading, not a three-dimensional measurement.

The World Health Organization definition finds bone mineral density and bone mineral content equal, or independently reliable, in predicting osteoporosis. But the prevalence of osteoporosis depends entirely upon the way in which DXA results are interpreted and expressed. For example, a United Kingdom study found that the prevalence of osteoporosis of the spine in women more than 70 years old has been found to be approximately 30 percent when measured in terms of BMD, but is only half that when BMC is used [20].

Dr. S. Pors Neilson discusses this in his article "The fallacy of BMD: a critical review of the diagnostic use of dual X-ray absorptiometry":

This fact is well known but is largely neglected. This neglect has the obvious consequence that osteoporosis is over-diagnosed in persons of petite body stature, simply because the means of reference populations are calculated from the values of large and small people [21].

In addition, the technical accuracy and precision of BMD measurements are considered by some to be barely satisfactory for clinical use. An accurate measurement would represent the true mineral content of the targeted bone site. But the error for DXA measurements can be up to 8 percent. This means that the true value of a woman's bone density could be 8 percent higher or lower than what is reported to her. That is equal to almost one standard deviation, enough to dramatically change her diagnosis [22].

Precision refers to whether the same bone site can be measured repeatedly with an identical outcome. In the absence of international standards, DXA machines are calibrated differently, so precision is far from guaranteed. For this reason it is important to always be measured using the same machine, using the same reference ranges, in follow-up testing.

A New Zealand "20/20" television documentary examined the issues surrounding osteoporosis. In a simple experiment, the producers sent Sally, a healthy 50-year-old woman, to be scanned by two different major brands of DXA machines in separate cities. Astoundingly she was only fractionally below normal on one DXA machine, but on the other had bone density so low that it was close to the threshold for a diagnosis of osteoporosis. In one clinic, she was given a clean bill of health, and in the other, she was advised to consider treatment.

And the same brand of machine can even produce different results on the same day! Dr. Susan Ott had 300 of her patients test their bone density twice: firstly when they arrived, and then again after walking about the room between measurements. She found that repeat measurements on the same day with the same machine can show as much as a 7 percent difference in bone mineral density [23].

Quantitative Ultrasound

Quantitative ultrasound offers a cheaper, more accessible method of bone density testing. It uses sound waves rather than X-rays, and most commonly measures the calcaneous or heel bone, as it is limited to bone with minimal overlying tissue. It is considered a reasonably useful diagnostic tool, but the results cannot be directly compared with the results of a DXA scan, which remains the industry standard. It is not fully understood exactly what is being measured with heel ultrasound. It appears to mainly measure bone density. A study of 149,524 postmenopausal women suggests that ultrasound and peripheral BMD testing may predict an increased risk for fracture. The study found that low BMD in the heel, forearm, or finger was associated with a two-fold increased risk for fracture within one year [24]. Still, this method of measuring bone density suffers from the same problems of classification that DXA scanning does — it classifies a large number of women at risk, many of whom will never experience a fracture.

Establishing Normal Peak Bone Mass

DXA measures the bone mineral density of an individual and then "grades" it against an average peak bone mass, or peak bone density, which has been established from a selected young reference population. But as researchers have found, peak bone mass varies widely from region to region, by gender, and even fluctuates seasonally. A Mexican survey of more than 4,000 healthy young people showed wide regional variations in peak bone density, and a Canadian study revealed similar inconsistencies [25]. Consequently, concerned scientists and osteoporosis experts are warning that the technology may be diagnosing "low bone density" when it is at a normal level for that person — a level that may never result in a fracture.

Peak Bone Mass Defined

Adolescence is a crucial time for bone development. Surges in growth and reproductive hormones initiate a spurt in bone growth that is responsible for almost half of the adult bone mass. Peak bone mass (PBM) usually occurs around age 20. It is the total bone mass or density that a young person has after they have completed the growth of their long bones. The level of peak bone mass achieved in any individual is the result of all the things that have happened to the skeleton from its formation in the uterus through the years of growth into young adulthood. It is the sum of genetic and environmental factors. Once peak bone mass is achieved, bone mass tends to remain stable in both males and females until their late 30s and 40s. After this time, it begins to decline, at different rates for different individuals, and at different rates for different sites in the body. Bone density is, on average, lower in women than in men, but there is a wide range among individuals. Women on average lose between one-third and one-half of their peak bone mass over their lifetime, while men lose less [26].

It is believed that genetic factors account for an estimated 60 percent to 80 percent of the variability in PBM, with diet, physical activity, and hormonal status being important factors as well [27]. Some bones will continue to grow. The skull increases in mass throughout life. Certain bones, the femur (thighbone) and vertebrae, for example, continue to increase in diameter, as we get older. It is generally agreed that the greater the peak bone mass achieved in youth, the greater protection a person has against fracture later in life when bone density progressively decreases for everyone. But this is only an assumption and doesn't account for normal variations in PBM and bone density. The natural history of bone development before menopause, and changes over a lifetime are particularly poorly understood because of a lack of longitudinal studies with good methodology and design.

Bone Physiology

In general, bone physiology is considered similar in males and females. Structurally, bone is of two types — trabecular bone and cortical bone. Trabecular bone is the more porous, honeycomb-like bone that forms the inner meshwork of the vertebrae, pelvis, flatbones and the ends of long bones. Trabecular bone constitutes 20 percent of the skeleton but has a large surface area and is sensitive to metabolic changes. Trabecular bone is the type of bone most subject to loss of density as we grow older, and to loss of structural integrity and strength with established osteoporosis.

Cortical, or compact bone, which makes up 80 percent of the skeleton, forms the outer casing of all bones and is the major constituent of the shaft of long bones. The loss of bone that occurs with aging results in up to 35 percent reduction of cortical bone and a 50 percent reduction of trabecular bone in women. Men lose approximately 25 percent and 35 percent of cortical and trabecular bone respectively. Interestingly, one study showed that males have larger bones, but not necessarily stronger bones. The trabecular bone density was the same in males and females, and decreased with age in both. Whether DXA scanning using women's criteria for diagnosis is relevant for men is under debate. Generally, the criteria established for women are applied in the same way to men.

Manufacturers' Reference Standards

When you have your bone density measured by a DXA machine, you are given a computerized analysis indicating whether your bone density is normal, above, or below normal. "Normal" is a level set in the software of the DXA machine. If you are more than one standard deviation below that, then you are classified as abnormal.

What people often don't realize is that they are not being compared to their own peak bone mass or to that of their own age group. Instead, they are being measured against that of a selected group of young "normal individuals," established by the DXA manufacturer. The WHO definition of osteoporosis recommends all women be measured and diagnosed using a young normal reference population. This is called a T-score. A Z-score is when you are measured against an average BMD for your age and gender, but this is not used to formally diagnose. Because everyone loses bone density as they age, using T-scores instead of Z-scores guarantees that almost all older women will fall into the "negative" range. Their normal age related bone loss will automatically be categorized as osteopenia or osteoporosis. If Z-scores were used, it is unlikely there would be an epidemic of osteoporosis.

Here is the surprising thing:

There is no agreed international reference standard, and each manufacturer has established its own independent, average young normal data, resulting in vastly different standards between brands of DXA machines.

The major manufacturers of DXA machines in the United States have created their young normal reference standards by measuring the peak bone mass of healthy, young white women of different ages. For one group, the age range was 20 to 29. For another, it was 20 to 39. One population included women up to the age of 50 years. One manufacturer reported that its reference data was obtained from 3,000 U.S. and Northern European females, 1,400 French females, and 1,400 Japanese females [28], while another drew its reference subjects from the University of California in San Diego. This latter population is not believed to be a random sample of the population — they were chosen because they were *exceptionally* healthy, so they do not represent a normal, young, healthy adult. Screening in this way can create an artificially high "normal" or mean peak bone mass, which inevitably leads to biased results. Under these conditions, many more people will be found to have low bone density and will consequently be given a diagnosis of osteoporosis [29].

During the course of their research, the authors of the British Columbia Technology Assessment review of the effectiveness of BMD testing contacted the manufacturers of DXA machines to find out how the "young normal" subjects were selected. Other than obvious reasons for exclusion, such as medication, substance abuse, and illness, they were given very little information about important factors like age, nutrition, exercise patterns, and even weight and height of the individuals. The authors of the study conclude: "We have no assurance that the range of 'young normals' were not biased by the inclusion of a disproportionately large number of athletic team members [30]."

More recently, concerned researchers in various countries have established their own young normal standards based on local populations. They have invariably found them to be different from the manufacturer's — usually much lower. When they have applied their own local reference standards for general screening instead of the manufacturer's, the outcomes have been very different. This suggests that massive variations in diagnosis are taking place — dependent entirely upon which country or which machine is doing the measuring.

Two large studies, one in the United States and one in Canada, measured local population samples of young people in order to set their own DXA reference standards. The studies then measured a large cross section of the population using their local standards and compared this with the manufacturer's standard. The first study, the third National Health and Nutrition Examination Survey (NHANES III), chose a sample of young women who were more diverse in terms of body size and other environmental factors than the manufacturer's group. For example, young women with pre-existing illnesses who were taking medications were not excluded, and although this was unlikely to affect bone loss, it meant that there was more variation in height and weight than in the healthy volunteers used by the manufacturers. Researchers did this to obtain a reference group that accurately reflects a normal average BMD level — one that actually exists in the population [31]. The result was an average peak bone mass that was much lower than the DXA companies'. This cut the prevalence of osteoporosis, as defined by BMD, by more than half. That is, if researchers had used the manufacturers' reference range in their study, the prevalence of osteoporosis of the hip would have been 49 percent, rather than the 28 percent they found [32].

The second study, a Canadian government-funded epidemiological study of 10,000 people, set its own population-specific reference standard using a random selection of young women. The results they came up with were equally astonishing. They found the actual prevalence of osteoporosis (as defined by low bone density) to be 16 percent in women and 5 percent in men, as opposed to the official Canadian estimates of 50 percent and 12 percent [33].

When the researchers of the Canadian study applied the NHANES III criteria for the hip and compared the results to the

Canadian criteria, the outcomes were similar. When they were compared with manufacturer's criteria, however, the outcome was vastly different.

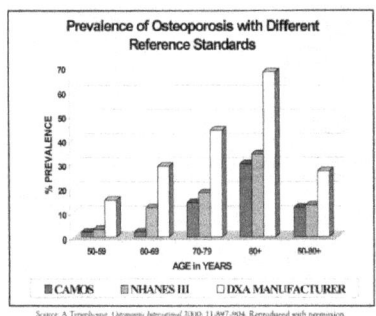

Estimation of the Prevalence of Low Bone Density in Canadian Women and Men Using a Population-Specific DXA Reference Standard

A study from Turkey shows the prevalence of low BMD fell from 50.3 percent to 14 percent at the spine, and from 60.8 percent to 14.6 percent at the hip, when the manufacturer's standard was compared with a locally produced standard [34]. The authors conclude: "... our data suggest that individual populations should use their own reference range T-scores in DXA in order to avoid misdiagnoses of osteopenia and osteoporosis based on other population's reference range T-scores. Since a low normal BMD is not necessarily indicative of an increased risk of fracture in a given population, this approach might decrease unnecessary patient anxiety and errors concerning treatment [35]."

In a study from the United Kingdom published in 1997, the bone mineral densities of 2,068 women aged 30 to 70 were measured. Fifty-four percent were in the normal range, according to a locally determined standard, but only 25 percent were normal against the manufacturer's standard, leading the researchers to comment: "We observe that manufacturer's reference ranges may not be appropriate for the local population and may lead to an erroneously high diagnosis of osteopenia and osteoporosis, which would lead to unnecessary patient anxiety and perhaps errors regarding treatment [36]."

Another U.K. study reports: "Our findings suggest that patients may be diagnosed as having osteoporosis if one reference range is used but not if another is used, even when the same manufacturer's dual-energy X-ray absorptiometry system is used [37]."

Not surprisingly, many experts have question the relevance and accuracy of current standards for DXA scanning and the WHO criteria [38,39 40]. Correcting the situation is not simple as updates or changes to overcome these major problems can make it very difficult to interpret previous readings [41].

Overall, doctors and general practitioners who recommend bone scanning to their patients are unaware of the controversy, and trustingly make decisions on the basis of the outcome of a DXA scan. The massive discrepancies in the diagnosis of osteoporosis, resulting from inconsistent and inaccurate DXA scanning, raise serious concerns. Many people are being diagnosed with osteoporosis and then treated with prescription medications, when they will never have a fragility fracture.

The Toll on the Patient

The psychological effects of being labeled abnormal or at risk are rarely considered. Such labels cause great distress and anxiety, and are known to "affect the identity and shape the life experience of those who are so labeled [42]." My years as a menopause educator have confirmed the prevailing fear many women have of developing osteoporosis. Their doctors routinely recommend BMD testing as part of the menopause "wellness" package. Once such testing is embarked upon, women are invariably caught in the re-screening loop. An abnormal diagnosis requires repeat testing, which leads to increasing dependency on BMD testing. Osteoporosis drugs are also likely to be administered over many years to ensure that women retain "normal" levels of bone density.

Susie looked very anxious as she told her story. She had an early menopause, used HRT for only a few months, and then managed the rather difficult transition with exercise and herbal treatments. Ten years later, at age 48, she had been recommended to undergo bone density testing because she was told her early menopause put her at greater risk for osteoporosis. Her bone density measured normal, but she was still worried.

Although her bone density was normal, it was at the low end of normal. Because Susie believed she was on the brink of rapid age-related bone loss, she thought the result meant she was still at serious risk for fracture. She could not be reassured. She was convinced by the information from her doctor and the computerized printout from the DXA machine that her bone mass was about to slip from the "normal" range into the "diseased" category.

Accuracy of diagnosis is imperative. Younger perimenopausal women who are identified as having low bone mass in the spine are likely to be encouraged to embark upon treatment, even there is little or no evidence for benefit in this group.

Postmenopausal women had previously reported that the results of bone densitometry testing substantially influenced their decision to begin treatment. A study found that women with moderate bone loss (osteopenia) were twice as likely to start treatment as women with normal bone density, and women with very low bone density (osteoporosis) were more than three times as likely to start, regardless of whether they had had a previous fragility fracture [43].

BMD Testing – Further Limitations

Bone mineral density testing has other limitations as well. The sites most commonly measured are the hip and the spine. But bone density can vary throughout the skeleton. It is hardly conclusive that you have osteoporosis when one part of you, for instance the lower spine, registers low bone density, because the hip may be normal, or vice versa. The NHANES III study found that even different parts of the hip resulted in vastly different measurements. For example, only 10 percent of the population studied had osteoporosis in the whole hip (femur) region, whereas 17 to 20 percent had osteoporosis when each region of the hip was considered separately. In one group of women, 17 percent would have been classified as having osteoporosis in terms of the WHO criteria after having just the neck of the femur scanned, but only 6 percent would have osteoporosis when the entire hip region was scanned [44].

In the same study, the bone densities of 351 women and 348 men, ranging from 21 to 93 years of age, were measured in 15 body sites — including the spine, hip, wrist, leg, head, pelvis and ribs. Results differed considerably from one site to another, and from men to women. The areas with the lowest BMD were the lumbar spine, the hip, and the wrist. The stage of life when the bone density for a given area was lost was quite different. Bone density in the hip, for example, began to decline very slowly from the age of 20, whereas spinal bone density was stable in women until menopause [45].

Perspective from Independent Analysts

Reports on bone mineral testing and associated treatments were furnished by 14 agencies for health technology assessment after the re-defining of osteoporosis. In 1996 the British Columbia Office of Health Technology Assessment analyzed findings of 14 major review groups and concluded that BMD testing does *not* result in a reduction of fractures and is therefore not a cost-effective public health strategy.

With regard to the evidence for national screening programs, the independent analysts had this to say:

The International Network of Agencies for Health Technology Assessment:
When all the scenarios are considered, a BMD screening program aimed at menopausal women might prevent between 1 percent and 7 percent of fractures. Taken together, these estimates of the effectiveness of such a program are not particularly encouraging from a public health perspective and are unlikely to represent good value for the money [46].

Effective Health Care Bulletin, U.K.:
It is likely that a bone screening program will lead to the prevention of no more than 5 percent of fractures in elderly women. Given the current evidence, it would be inadvisable to establish a routine population-based bone screening program for menopausal women with the aim of preventing fractures [47].

The substantial concerns raised by health technology assessment agencies on the effectiveness of bone density measurement and associated treatments were not listened to at the time. In recent years they have been proven right. But not before millions of women worldwide were diagnosed with a condition they didn't have, and proceeded to take HRT and then bisphosphonates long term to prevent future disease, exposing themselves to unaccountable dangers.

A Salutary Tale

The British Columbia Medical Services Commission imposed a moratorium on public funding of bone densitometry (DXA) testing, following the release of the 1996 report by the BC Office of Health Technology Assessment that called into question the effectiveness of bone density screening. This stopped the growth of BMD technology in publicly funded facilities in the province for three years. The medical consultant who chaired the British Columbia Ministry of Health at the time was responsible for the moratorium; he was convinced that there was no scientific evidence that BMD testing led to better patient outcomes. In 1999, the medical consultant's contract was not renewed, and he left the ministry. The BMD moratorium ended, and in 1999 the number of publicly funded facilities with BMD-testing capacity doubled. Commercial interests quickly resumed, promoting BMD testing in the province [48].

Ken Bassett, a member of the BCOHTA group, pays tribute to the medical consultant's decision and its consequences, and warns: "Its outcome reminds us … about the power and persistence of the private interests whose well-being depends on selling tests and drugs, whatever the evidence might indicate, and of the daunting challenge of attempting to forestall the diffusion of technology that has gained a foothold [49]."

Other Screening Methods

Bone Remodeling and Bone Markers

Bone is a living organ that is constantly remodeling, replacing, and repairing itself. The adult skeleton is replaced entirely every seven to 10 years. From birth to adolescence and, to a lesser degree, young adulthood, there is massive bone remodeling as we grow taller and the long bones continue to extend. After the adolescent growth period ceases, the bone remodeling process slows, entering the maintenance phase. Then, after menopause, most women appear to have higher levels of bone remodeling once again, although this can vary. In men, the age-related thinning of bones seems to occur about 10 years later than it does in women.

The process of remodeling serves two purposes. First, it keeps bones "young." When you knock your leg or strain to lift a heavy object, the area of bone that bears the impact will begin to repair the micro-damage that has occurred. Second, remodeling makes bone better able to meet the demands placed upon it. This is why a violinist's bow arm, a TV cameraman's holding arm, or a tennis player's racquet arm, all develop bone that is thicker and stronger than the bone of the arm that is less used [50].

During the bone remodeling process, certain chemical by-products are produced which can be found in blood and urine. Different chemicals are produced during the bone formation and resorption. These chemicals, called bone markers, have become a relatively new addition to the osteoporosis diagnosis field. By measuring an individual's bone markers, researchers can better gauge if a person's bone resorption is too high or formation is too low, and if treatment is embarked upon, can give some indication of its success after two or three months.

While the accuracy of biochemical markers of bone turnover has improved markedly in the past few years, there is still debate about their application. The general consensus is that measurement of bone turnover markers provides potentially useful information to supplement BMD measurement, but cannot be used to diagnose osteoporosis, evaluate its severity, or select a specific therapy.

Bone Resorption and Formation Markers

Bone is the only organ that has cells designed specifically to destroy it. They are called *osteoclasts*. There are also cells called *osteoblasts*, whose sole purpose is to repair the organ. Healthy bones remodel and repair themselves in much the same way that road maintenance crews repair damaged or weakened roads. Bone is like a well-used highway, which becomes cracked and worn with use and will eventually crumble, unless the cracked and worn patches are removed and replaced. Bone remodeling occurs at sites where damage has occurred as a result of force, as in a knock or fall, or when muscles have been working hard, applying great pressure to bone. Breaking or cracking a bone generates an awe-inspiring sequence of events, which results in complete repair and new, well formedbone tissue. A certain amount of muscle strain also helps to maintain bone. That is why exercise, particularly weight-bearing, is essential to perpetuate healthy bone remodeling.

The bone maintenance crews are called BMUs (basic multi-cellular units). About one million of these crews are working to remove and replace bone at any one time. When damage occurs in a patch of bone, it is sensed by a network of cells called *osteocytes*, which send signal molecules to alert the BMUs via an extensive "osteo-internet." As in road repair, the first members of the BMU to arrive are the diggers, the osteoclasts, which begin their process of removing damaged bone. This process is known as resorption.

As the osteoclasts dig out the damaged patch, they actually release bone growth-triggering factors that were left there two to five years earlier by cells called osteoblasts, whose purpose it is to rebuild the bone. These factors stimulate new osteoblasts to begin the rebuilding process. The osteoclasts dig tunnels and trenches at the rate of about 1,000th of an inch per day. Osteoblasts secrete collagen and laboriously fill in the excavated areas, but take about eight times longer to do so. Gradually, the new bone mineralizes around the new web of collagen and, after about six to nine months, the process is complete.

At certain times of life, there is more bone building than remodeling — as in childhood and youth — so osteoblast cells predominate. Although the full story is not known, it seems that as we age, the BMUs are not as effective at patching and maintaining bone, and we begin to lose more bone than we gain. It is believed that reduced bone density and osteoporosis occur when many factors combine to produce BMUs with deeper-digging osteoclasts and smaller crews of osteoblasts that cannot fill the bigger holes.

Resorption Markers

1. Dpd

As the bone is broken down, a substance called deoxypyridinoline, or Dpd, is excreted in the urine. Dpd is the product of a type of collagen found in bones and is a specific marker of bone breakdown; its levels are unaffected by diet, making it suitable for assessing resorption.

Because bones remodel at a higher rate

while people sleep, Dpd is measured from a urine sample collected from the first or second urination in the morning. A Dpd score of less than 6.5nM/mM is considered normal in some labs, based on the levels for healthy men and premenopausal women who are not pregnant. A high Dpd measurement, for adults who are past their bone-growing years, indicates that bone is being lost. Whether the bone-loss rate is cause for alarm is another issue. It is not known whether the Dpd test can predict risk for fracture.

2. Collagen Cross-links (NTX, CTX)
The activity of osteoclasts is measured by breakdown products of collagen. When bone is resorbed, collagen is broken down and fragments that contain the cross-linking molecules are released and excreted in the urine. High levels can indicate high levels of bone resorption.

Formation Markers

1. Bone Alkaline Phosphatase (ALP)
Osteoblastic activity, or bone formation, is associated with osteocalcin, one of the proteins found in relatively high

concentrations in bone. Bone alkaline phosphatase (ALP) forms new calcium crystals, and blood levels of this bone enzyme give an indication of new bone formation. However, alkaline phosphatase is formed by many of the body's tissues. Therefore, the routine reporting of ALP levels on liver function tests does not give any information about *bone* alkaline phosphatase. For this, further testing is required.

2. *Propeptide of Type 1 Collagen (PICP)*
Bone is made up of a framework or matrix of interlocking fibers of the protein collagen, which forms the foundation for bone structure, and inorganic components that surround the collagen structure and form the "cement." Collagen is normally flexible and is important in the structure of skin and nails. In bone, however, it is made strong and rigid by tiny crystals of calcium phosphate salts. This test measures PICP, which is associated with the secretion of collagen. It has been shown to correlate with bone formation.

Diagnostic Methods in Perspective

The connection between bone formation and resorption is poorly understood at present. It is a key puzzle to be solved in the field of bone biology. When a woman is identified with low bone density, it does not automatically mean that she has reduced bone formation and greater bone resorption. Young people can have low bone density, and older people can have higher bone density [51].

None of these testing methods gives an accurate assessment of bone strength. Because of the great variability in bone turnover, the seasonal variation of bone density, and the day-to-day variation of metabolic processes, these tests cannot accurately assess the risk of future bone fracture.

The Doctor's Dilemma

Women accept the advice of their doctors, believing them to be fully informed about the accuracy of methods for diagnosing osteoporosis, and the effectiveness and safety of treatments. Unfortunately, most physicians are not well informed. Authors of the Alberta Technology Assessment Review comment that the significance and limitations of BMD results seem poorly understood in general practice [52].

Concerns have also been raised about the interpretation of BMD results. Knowledge of statistics is required, and interpretations can vary from one laboratory and physician to another. A person with osteoporosis can be cared for by her general practitioner, gynecologist, endocrinologist, or a rheumatologist, each with a unique approach to assessing the condition.

The dilemma for physicians is to determine whether low bone density puts their patient at risk for fracture, and therefore whether to recommend treatment. Most doctors are not aware that evidence linking low BMD to fracture is minimal, and that they may do their patient greater harm by prescribing medication. It is hard to argue with the apparent objectivity of a machine.

***

Chapter 4
The Myth of Causality

Myth #3: Age-related bone loss is the cause of deadly fractures in the elderly.

Ruth, at the age of 82, underwent DXA scanning at the request of her primary care physician. Her results for the lumbar spine were in the osteoporosis range and for the hip the osteopenia range. She was advised to start taking Fosamax. After reading about the side effects of the drug, she wanted a second opinion. She consulted a physician who showed her a study from the New England Journal of Medicine. Citing the article, the doctor informed Ruth that she had no risk factors for osteoporosis other than her age and her low bone density results. Even though her hipbonedensity was in the range of osteopenia, it was average for women her age. (Her lumbar spine bone density was just below average for her age.) The doctor showed her that even if the drug could improve her bone density from average to the highest third, her risk of a hip fracture would not decrease. She decided not to take the drug.

Like many people, Ruth was concerned about osteoporosis and was afraid of sustaining a fracture, though she had little information about her bone health — other than a measurement of low bone density. This is because physicians and researchers continue to emphasize the single risk factor of low bone density. The concern about osteoporosis, however, is really a concern about fractures. If bone thinned with aging but no one ever fractured, osteoporosis would be an obscure academic subject reserved for the medical texts. Understanding fractures and what causes them is the key issue.

Fractures related to bone fragility tend to occur at sites containing a higher percentage of the porous, honeycomb-like trabecular bone — the predominant bone type in the hip and spine. Other sites that may have fragility fractures are the wrist and the ribs. Fractures of the skull, ankle, and the long bones of the leg are not usually associated with osteoporosis fractures [1].

Like so many processes, functions and conditions in the human body, the causes of fractures are complex. Attributing fractures to low bone density alone is an oversimplification.

Hip Fractures

The hype surrounding hip fractures can be frightening; especially the chilling mantra that around 25 percent of people who fracture a hip will be dead within 6 months or a year. In reality, although it may be the 'last straw' for an elderly very frailperson, healthy women rarely die from hip fractures. Routine modern hip replacement procedures have individuals up and walking often within days. In women who were mobile before a hip or pelvic fracture, it is estimated that as few as 14 percent of their deaths were caused or hastened by the fractures [2].

A 50-year-old woman has a 15 percent likelihood of fracturing a hip in her lifetime and a man has a 5 percent to 6 percent chance [3]. Among men and women who live to the age of 90, 32 percent of females and 17 percent of males will have a hip fracture [4]. Hip fractures occur after a fall — even though only 1 percent of all falls in the elderly result in a fracture. The direction of the fall plays a large role in the outcome. A fall to the side, as opposed to forward or backward, increases the risk of hip fracture by about six times, and is considered a much greater risk than lower bone density [5].

Dr. Susan Ott, osteoporosis expert, comments: "Other factors include how tall a patient is, how far she falls, how she lands, and maybe the shape of her hip. Also, factors that cannot be measured may be involved, such as how many of the bone cells are alive, how brittle the bone itself is, etc [6]."

The National Institutes of Health writes:

Fracture risk has been consistently associated with a history of falls, low physical function such as slow gait speed and decreased quadriceps strength, impaired cognition, impaired vision, and the presence of environmental hazards (e.g., throw rugs) [7].

A British study concludes that the following factors were more accurate than low BMD in predicting hip fracture in the elderly: low body weight, kyphosis, poor circulation in the foot, epilepsy, short-term use of steroids, and poor trunk maneuverability [8].

Many of the conditions that increase the likelihood of a person falling (and breaking a hip) can be symptoms of advanced age: poor eyesight; weakened balance coordination and strength; and confused mind (often the result of medication side effects).

Mental health also plays an important role. A British study found that patients with depression, dementia, or delirium appeared to be at increased risk of death after hip fracture. Dr. John Holmes from the University of Leeds conducted the study and concluded that the "findings confirm what is not widely appreciated: that psychiatric illnesses have important effects on physical conditions [9]."

The healthier a woman is, the less likely she is to fall and break her hip. And the healthier a person is prior to a hip fracture, the better the chance of a good recovery.

To put a positive slant on it, 85 percent of women aged 50 with a life expectancy of 80 years will *not* suffer a hip fracture.

Mechanical Factors

At least half of all of hip fractures after the age of 80 are linked to mechanical factors, not bone fragility. Common cervical fractures, or fractures of the femoral neck, appear to be more related to pelvic structure than osteoporosis — that is, failure of the outer diameter of the femoral neck to expand with age and increased acetabular bone width. Women with trochanteric hip fractures (the wider area of bone at the head of the femur) have a more severe and generalized bone loss due to the greater amount of trabecular bone in that region of the hip [10]. Overall, about half of hip fractures are intertrochanteric, and the others are femoral neck fractures. In older women the proportion of trochanteric fractures increases.

Hip fracture is influenced by how weight on the hip is loaded, and of structural features as hip axis length. Many of these aspects vary across cultures. For example, hip fracture risk doubles with each standard deviation increase in hip axis length. Asian adults have shorter hip axes than adult Caucasians;

consequently, Asians have a lower hip fracture risk [11].

Multiple risk factors to predict fracture

A study of 9,516 white women over the age of 65 measured the risk factors for hip fracture. The following are listed as the most predictive factors:

* A maternal history of hip fracture

* Having the same body weight as at age 25

* Previous fractures after the age of 50

* Being tall at the age of 25

* Self-rated health being fair or poor

* Previous hyperthyroidism

* Medications — specifically sedatives, antidepressants and long-acting benzodiazepines or anticonvulsant drugs

* Less than four hours a day on feet [12]

Women who had five or more risk factors, including low bone density in the heel, were more likely to have a hip fracture than women who had no more than two risk factors, regardless of bone density [13]. The authors conclude that maintaining body weight, walking for exercise, avoiding medications with harmful side effects, minimizing caffeine intake, and treating impaired visual function are among steps that may decrease risk.

An Australian study found that a history of smoking, being underweight in old age and being overweight at age 20 were linked to an increased risk for hip fracture. Consumption of dairy products, particularly at age 20, was associated with an *increased* risk of hip fracture in older age. The authors conclude that older people can reduce their risk of hip fracture by being reasonably physically active, maintaining a reasonable body weight, and stopping smoking [14].

The presence of a spine fracture or deformity is considered an important predictor of further fracture. The number of previous vertebral fractures along with low bone density is linked to a greater risk for vertebral fractures, while the severity of previous vertebral fractures alone is the risk factor that predicts non-vertebral (such as hip) fractures [15].

Hip Pads

In elderly people who are at high risk for fracture, the wearing of a padded undergarment can help prevent such an event. The undergarment incorporates a soft, thin pad over each hipbone and works similarly to the padding in a football player's uniform. The hip pad absorbs the shock of a fall, disperses its impact over a larger area, and reduces the force of a fall on the vulnerable hip. A recent study found that the frail at-risk group who wore the underwear experienced five times as many falls as the healthier control group — though the at-risk group sustained no fractures. The control group had a 4.3 percent fracture rate [16].

Despite the effectiveness of the undergarments, they are not widely promoted by doctors. In addition, many elderly people prefer not to wear them because they find them uncomfortable and bulky. A United Kingdom study of 153 residents of residential care homes found that only 3 percent of people would wear them at night and that daytime compliance rates reduced from 47 percent for the first month, to around 30 percent for months five and six [17].

Vertebral Fractures

Vertebrae tend to compress or become deformed when bone tissue deteriorates with age. Most vertebral deformities occur without any associated pain or major symptoms and 'fractures' are revealed when found incidentally by X-ray. Fractures of the vertebrae range from mild to severe. Vertebrae do not usually break as such, so fracture may be a misleading term. Researchers determine vertebral fractures by measuring the height and width of individual vertebra and comparing them to reference ranges. Although criteria vary, if the height of a given vertebra has decreased by more than 3 standard deviations (or 20 percent to 25 percent), it is generally deemed a fracture [18].

The wedging of vertebrae that causes curvature in the spine can occur normally to some degree with aging and is not necessarily associated with marked bone loss or fragility [19]. Loss of height may occur suddenly or gradually and is commonly due to thinning of the cartilage discs between the vertebrae.

The spine consists of 24 vertebrae, each one cushioned by a flat, cylindrical disk made from cartilage. The larger flat bone at the bottom of the vertebrae is called the sacrum, and the tiny tailbone underneath, the coccyx.

The spine is divided into three sections:

The cervical spine: the seven vertebrae at the top of the spine that are generally less likely to be affected by osteoporosis.

The thoracic spine: the 12 vertebrae in the middle of the back that have a pair of ribs attached to each of them. These bones are more prone to abnormality. It is a wedge fracture in the thoracic spine that can form the spinal "hump."

The lumbar spine: the five vertebrae below the thoracic region. These vertebrae are also susceptible to abnormalities.

DXA scanning technology is not precise enough to identify spinal deformity. This can only be determined with X-ray and careful assessment. Even then, the degree of compression of the vertebra necessary to define an actual vertebral fracture is not standardized. (A height loss of more than 4 centimeters over 10 years has been used as a measure to determinethat a vertebral fracture has occurred.) There is continued controversy in the osteoporosis community over what actually constitutes a vertebral fracture.

Clinical vertebral compression fractures may be very painful. The pain generally lasts a few months and can be managed with bed rest and analgesics. The fracture will heal, and normal life and activities can be resumed [20].

In rare, serious cases, the vertebrae become wedge-shaped and an elderly woman may develop a hump in her back after multiple wedge fractures. This is called a dowager's hump and can bring chronic pain and other complications. The image of the hunched-over woman with the dowager's hump has been frequently used in advertising — often with the effect of scaring the women who see such images — but just how common is the condition? An Australian study of fragility fractures cites the lifetime risk of multiple spinal fractures as 3 percent [21].

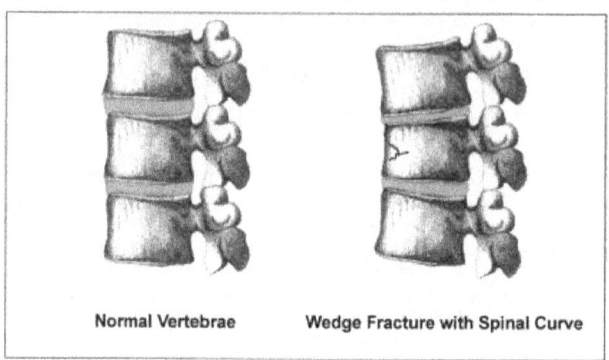

Normal Vertebrae   Wedge Fracture with Spinal Curve

Confusing Statistics

Because there is no international standard for defining the degree of compression necessary to establish a vertebral fracture, there is wide variability in rates of fracture.

Dr. Susan Ott comments: "With vertebral fractures the incidence depends on how you measure the vertebra. If you define a fracture as only a small decrease in height, then there will be a lot of them. If you use stricter criteria, then there are not as many. Several good studies have recently been reported showing how much difference it can make [22]."

And even when the same criteria for defining a vertebral fracture are applied, the rates vary widely from one location to the next. In Europe for example, the prevalence of deformities of the vertebrae shows enormous variation from country to country — as much as from 6 to 20 percent [23]. The highest rates are in Scandinavian countries.

To put the incidence of vertebral fracture in perspective, Dr. Bruce Ettinger, osteoporosis expert, writes:

Clinical vertebral fractures are rare — vertebral deformities based on careful radiographic assessments are much more common. The incidence of the latter [deformities] is about 1 in 200 to 1 in 300 women per year. Clinical fractures are about 1/3 of this rate. The 10 year risk of painful spine fracture for women at age 50 or at age 60 is very low, but the rate increases quite a bit with aging [24].

Treatments For Vertebral Fractures

Bisphosphonates and other drugs are routinely prescribed but the benefits and risks must be carefully considered. (See Chapter 6)

Two procedures, vertebroplasty and kyphoplasty, have been developed to manage the pain of acute vertebral fractures. They are procedures where bone cement is injected through a small hole in the skin into a fractured vertebra. The procedures are controversial with conflicting evidence regarding their effectiveness. There is a risk of a leak of the acrylic cement outside of the vertebral body. Although severe complications are rare, infection, bleeding, numbness, tingling, headache, and paralysis may ensue due to misplacement of the needle or cement. When the cement has leaked into blood vessels, heart and lung damage and some deaths have occurred. A 2009 study found no benefit from vertebroplasty [25].

Wrist Fractures

Fractures of the wrist are common in women 50 to 70 years old — the age when a woman's balance begins to decline, which can result in a fall. Wrists break when women fall and stretch out their arms to brace themselves. This tends to cause a fracture in the wrist at the end of one of the two bones in the forearm (the radius). This type of fracture is called a Colles' fracture. While other bones in the wrist may fracture, Colle's fractures are the most common. A white woman has a 15 percent chance of fracturing her wrist during her lifetime.

As a woman ages further, her reaction time declines; when she falls she is unable to brace herself and is more likely to fall directly onto her hip, rather than on her outstretched arms. Fitness, agility, and speed of gait are also factors. Women who walk faster are more likely to have forward momentum, and if they fall, they land on their wrists.

A Colles' fracture can occur with normal, high, or low bone density of the forearm [26]. Research indicates that factors related to bone geometry rather than bone density are linked to forearm fractures [27]. Wrist fractures, although painful, usually repair successfully. They do not typically have a long-term effect on a woman's quality of life. Neither do they predict subsequent fractures of the hip or spine. They cannot be described as debilitating or devastating, and hardly warrant long-term drug therapy as a preventative measure. To date there is no evidence that current medications will prevent wrist fracture. In fact Fosamax trials have shown a higher rate of wrist fracture with those on the treatment compared to placebo [28].

Secondary Causes of Osteoporosis

In many cases, an underlying medical condition contributes to the loss of bone and bone strength. A diagnosis of severely low bone density may indicate that some other condition, disease, or disorder is behind it and may increase a person's likelihood of fracture. These are known as secondary causes.

In pre- and peri-menopausal women, more than 50 percent of osteoporosis diagnoses are associated with secondary causes, the most common being glucocorticoid drugs (steroids that are prescribed for conditions ranging from asthma to arthritis); thyroid hormone excess; antiepileptic therapy; and low estrogen levels - often the result of surgical removal of the ovaries [29].

In cases where young people fracture easily and have low bone mass, there is commonly a secondary cause such as eating disorders or menstrual irregularities due to over-exercising. Those who take prednisone and other glucocorticoids are also at risk, as these medications are known to weaken bone. The U.S. National Institutes of Health have called for the development of glucocorticoids that will not adversely affect the skeleton [30].

In postmenopausal women, the prevalence of secondary conditions is thought to be lower. However, in one study of postmenopausal women, researchers identified several factors that contributed to the loss of bone, including hypercalciuria, (the excretion of abnormally large amounts of calcium in the urine), hyperparathyroidism (the over production of parathyroid hormone by the parathyroid glands), and malabsorption (poor absorption of nutrients via the digestive system). These women were found to have low bone mineral density [31].

Osteoporosis in men is usually related to secondary causes such as alcoholism, hypogonadism, and glucocorticoid treatments for asthma, rheumatoid arthritis, inflammations, and other ailments [32]. Studies estimate that 30 to 60 percent of osteoporosis in men is associated with secondary causes. Testosterone, like estrogen, is implicated in bone loss. Testosterone increases muscle mass, which indirectly results in higher bone density.

A study of 355 men more than 60 years old revealed several secondary causes which contributed to lower bone density, including: previous fractures, gastrectomy, peptic ulcer disease, rheumatoid arthritis, glucocorticoid use, hypertension, previous hyperthyroidism, height loss since age 20, chronic lung disease, and smoking [33].

Medical Conditions

A number of medical conditions are associated with lowered bone density and increased risk of fracture:

* hormone disorders such as hyperparathyroidism, hyperthyroidism, hypothyroidism
* gastrointestinal diseases such as celiac disease

* cystic fibrosis
* blood disorders
* genetic disorders
* connective tissue disease such as rheumatoid arthritis
* nutritional deficiencies
* a variety of other common serious chronic systemic disorders, such as congestive heart failure, end-stage renal disease, and alcoholism.

Drugs

A major factor for people at risk for osteoporosis is prescription drugs. The list of drugs which cause bone loss includes: steroids such as glucocorticoids, medroxyprogesterone acetate (Depo-Provera), heparin, alcohol, antacids, anti-seizure medications, cyclosporine A, exchange resins, lithium, luteinizing hormone-releasing hormone agonists, methotrexate, neuroleptics used to treat schizophrenia, and thyroid hormone (excess) [34].

Glucocorticoids (Corticosteroids)

Glucocorticoid use is the most common form of drug-related osteoporosis. The steroid is widely used for long-term disorders such as rheumatoid arthritis and other connective tissue diseases, asthma, psoriasis, Crohn's disease, lung disease, inflammatory bowel diseases, severe allergic reactions and inflammations, obstructive pulmonary disease, and in organ transplants. Corticosteroid treatment causes bone loss by a variety of complex mechanisms. Within the first year after starting corticosteroid therapy, patients lose on average 14 percent of their bone mineral content. Up to 50 percent of patients using the drug may fracture, especially postmenopausal women [35].

Patients treated with 10 milligrams of the corticosteroid prednisone for just 20 weeks experienced an 8 percent loss of BMD in the spine. High dose treatment (greater than the average daily dose of 7.5 milligrams of prednisone) has been shown to increase a patient's risk of developing vertebral fractures more than four-fold and to double the risk of experiencing a hip fracture. Even lower daily doses of corticosteroids (between 2.5 milligrams and 7.5 milligrams) have *been found to increase the risk of vertebral fractures 2.5 times. In addition, these lower-doses increase a patient's risk of developing a hip fracture by more than 75 percent [36].*

Patients who receive orally administered glucocorticoids (such as prednisone or cortisol) in a dose of 5 milligrams or more for longer than two months are at high risk for excessive bone loss. People who have undergone organ transplant are at high risk for osteoporosis due to a variety of factors, including pre-transplant organ failure and use of glucocorticoids after transplantation. The long-term effects on bone of intermittent use of systemic steroids or the chronic use of inhaled steroids, as are often used in asthma, are not known [37].

Depo-Provera (Medroxyprogesterone Acetate)

Depo-Provera is a contraceptive injection usually given every three months and also commonly used to treat premenstrual syndrome (PMS), pelvic pain syndrome, endometriosis, and advanced breast cancer in premenopausal women. It has been found to reduce bone density in young women by up to 4.1 percent per year, although bone density increases again once the treatment is stopped. Concerns have been raised about women using the drug around menopause, when bone density is naturally decreasing and is unlikely to recover in the same way as it does in a younger person when the treatment stops [38].

Heparin
Continued use in high doses of the blood-thinning drug heparin is associated with reduced bone density and osteoporosis-related fracture. Warfarin, another anticoagulant, has not been reported to have these effects [39].

Antacids
Taking large doses of antacids can cause severe bone pain, rickets (osteomalacia), and fractures. Stopping the treatment will rapidly improve symptoms.

Thyroid Hormone (L-Thyroxine) Replacement Therapy
Several studies have shown that long-term thyroxine therapy given to women with hypothyroidism may decrease bone

density, particularly in postmenopausal women [40].

Vitamin D Deficiency

Vitamin D, sometimes called a hormone and sometimes a nutrient, helps to control the formation of bone tissue. It increases the amount of calcium and phosphorus the body absorbs from the small intestine and thus helps regulate the growth, hardening, and repair of the bones.

Many adults, particularly those at the highest risk for fracture, have evidence of vitamin D deficiency. In states of vitamin D deficiency only a fraction of dietary calcium is absorbed, leading to accelerated bone loss, and increased risk for fracture. A 2005 review found vitamin D deficiency to be as high as 86 percent among older women in rest homes. The review also found that vitamin D deficiency was present in up to 76 percent of women with osteoporosis and 50 - 70 percent of women with a history of fracture [41].

A deficiency may also be linked to muscle weakness and bone pain, as it appears that adequate levels of vitamin D can preserve muscle strength and aid neuromuscular coordination. In a meta-analysis of 5 randomized trials involving a total of 1237 participants, vitamin D supplements in doses greater than 700 IU daily reduced the risk for falling by 22 percent compared with calcium or placebo [42]. (Read more about vitamin D in Chapter 6).

Thyroid Conditions

The thyroid gland, located in the neck below the Adam's apple area, regulates metabolism. It secretes hormones to help cells convert oxygen and calories into energy. A woman faces a 1-in-5 chance of developing thyroid problems during her lifetime. That risk increases with age and a family history of thyroid problems. Women may suffer from hyper (too much) or hypo (too little) thyroid hormones. Hyperthyroidism, an excess of circulating thyroid hormone, is a well-known risk factor for osteoporosis. Too much thyroid hormone increases metabolism to the point where more bone is destroyed than is created. Hyperthyroidism affects about 2 percent of women and 0.2 percent of men. Treatment for hyperthyroidism often involves surgery or ablation of the gland with radioactive iodine. Both procedures can result in hypothyroidism. There is evidence that women taking thyroid replacement medication for hypothyroidism may be at increased risk for excess bone loss, suggesting that careful regulation of thyroid replacement is important [43].

Hyperparathyroidism

Though the names are similar, the thyroid and parathyroid glands are separate glands, each producing distinct hormones with specific functions. The parathyroid glands are four pea-sized glands located on the thyroid gland in the neck. They secrete parathyroid hormone (PTH which helps maintain the correct balance of calcium and phosphorous in the body. PTH regulates release of calcium from bone, absorption of calcium in the intestine, and excretion of calcium in the urine. When the amount of calcium in the blood falls too low, the parathyroid glands secrete just enough PTH to restore the balance.

If the glands secrete too much hormone, as in hyperparathyroidism, the balance is disrupted and blood calcium rises. This condition of excessive calcium in the blood, (called hypercalcemia) or in the urine (hypercalciuria) indicates that something may be wrong with the parathyroid glands. Excess PTH triggers the release of too much calcium into the bloodstream. As a result, the bones may lose calcium, and too much calcium may be absorbed from food. The levels of calcium may increase in the urine causing kidney stones. PTH also acts to lower blood phosphorous levels by increasing excretion of phosphorus in the urine.

Menstrual Irregularities in Young Women

Failure to achieve peak bone mass, bone loss, and increased fracture rates have been evident in young women who have abnormal patterns of menstruation. Low levels of female hormones in a young woman brought about by delayed start of menstruation, very few menstrual periods, or an absence of menstrual periods are relatively common in adolescent girls and young women. These can occur as a result of strenuous athletic training, emotional stress, and low body weight.

Eating Disorders

Anorexia nervosa and bulimia are conditions that particularly affect young people, and can have devastating consequences. They usually involve an abnormal fear of obesity, a distorted body image, and abnormal eating patterns such as obsessive fasting, self-induced vomiting, or the use of laxatives. The effects of these disorders range from mild weight loss to delayed sexual development, heart problems, depression, osteoporosis, and even death.

Research has indicated that the condition might result in bone mass loss in up to 90 percent of anorexic women. Tests of 130 young women with anorexia showed that 38 percent of them had osteoporosis as defined by bone mineral density. Researchers from Massachusetts General Hospital indicated that 92 percent of the women showed bone mass loss at the hip, the spine and the extremities. The research indicated that supplementary female hormones (HRT) did not reduce the risk of bone mass loss in these women [44]. The investigators conclude that in these women body weight, not estrogen deficiencyis a significant predictor of bone mineral density, and stress that anorexic women should be counseled about the adverse effects of low weight on the skeleton [45].

In a statement from Massachusetts General Hospital, Boston, Dr. Anne Klibanski, one of the principal researchers says: "Some of these young women are experiencing bone loss comparable to that of women many decades older, despite estrogen therapy. Given this severity and the prevalence of bone loss, the importance of screening all women with anorexia for osteoporosis cannot be over-emphasized."

Celiac Disease

Celiac disease is a genetic disorder of the small bowel or the duodenum. The digestive tract is damaged by gluten proteins from wheat and other grains and is unable to effectively absorb nutrients including essential minerals for healthy bones. Celiac disease can account for a spectrum of illnesses ranging from relatively mild digestive symptoms to more serious conditions including osteoporosis, anemia, and diabetes. It is often undiagnosed because of its many mild and varied symptoms. Celiac disease can be simply and effectively reversed with the adoption of a gluten-free diet.

A large US study reported that approximately one in 133 Americans has the condition but maintains that only one out of 4,700 Americans has been diagnosed, causing 97 percent of cases go undetected [46]. Because many physicians don't consider celiac disease in determining a cause for osteoporosis, it is reasonable to conclude that a correctable cause of low bone density is being overlooked. In an Italian study, 86 newly diagnosed celiac disease patients, 66 percent of whom were found to have osteoporosis (low BMD) or osteopenia, adopted a gluten-free diet and then had their bones scanned again after one year. The gluten-free diet led to significant improvement in bone mineral density, even in postmenopausal women [47].

Other Causes

Cystic fibrosis and inflammatory bowel disease are examples of conditions associated with malabsorption and resultant low bone density in some individuals. Cystic fibrosis is also linked to the frequent need for corticosteroids as well as to other undefined factors.

The Myth of Causality

Low bone density is one of many risk factors for fracture, and often a minor one. The focus on low bone density has led to the myth that age-related bone loss is the major cause of fracture. In many cases, eliminating other risk factors and secondary causes of bone loss can do more to prevent fracture than attempting to increase bone density through medication. The excessive attention to low bone density has shifted the focus from modifiable risk factors to drug therapies. These therapies, discussed in the following chapters, come with their own set of concerns and problems.

***

SECTION II: TREATMENT MYTHS

***

Chapter 5
Overview of Drug Treatments

My eldest sister (now in her 60s) is one of millions of women who have been diagnosed with osteoporosis. Her bone density is low, and she has been strongly encouraged to take the bisphosphonate drug Fosamax long term. She has no vertebral fractures and hasn't fractured since she was 7 years old. She has no other risk factors for osteoporosis. She writes: "When I was first diagnosed with osteopenia prior to menopause [in 1996], I felt in a state of shock. The DXA scans showed I was well below the average, and I was told it was likely my bone density would reduce even further after menopause. My doctor wanted to prescribe hormone replacement therapy [HRT], but I didn't want to take it."

Barbara's doctor believed that HRT would slow down her bone density loss as she went through menopause and reduce her risk for fracture later. She had reservations about using HRT because she had heard conflicting reports about its safety. We now know she was right to trust her instincts. Evidence for serious risks associated with HRT means that long-term use for the prevention or treatment of osteoporosis is no longer advised.

The Case for Current Osteoporosis Treatments

My sister went for another bone density scan after menopause.

"Some years later another DXA scan had shown further lowering of my bone density particularly in the lower spine, and in addition to suggesting HRT, my physician also recommended the bisphosphonate Fosamax as a treatment option. He said there was 'a clear case for one or the other.' Feeling bolder after having refused to take HRT, I had arrived at the appointment with a folder of notes and a clipboard with my sheet of questions. I proceeded to take notes as he answered my questions, pausing and checking with him to make sure I had understood what he meant. At one stage, he leaned over

his desk, took my paper, and wrote the name of the drug we were discussing on my paper. 'FOSAMAX.' At the time, I felt his action intrusive and patronizing. It was a gesture I have not forgotten. An expert was telling me I had a serious condition that required what sounded like drastic long-term treatment, when I felt perfectly healthy. In addition, I knew by then that there were major questions around the effects and the value of this treatment."

Making the decision to embark on osteoporosis treatment is complex and difficult. The decision to undergo treatment must involve a careful weighing up of the risk for fracture against the risk of embarking on a treatment that cannot guarantee prevention of fracture and carries known and unknown long-term side effects. Sometimes drugs can appear to be more effective than they really are. Understanding the basics of medical terminology can prevent misunderstandings.

How significant is 'significant'?

When treatments claim to significantly increase bone density or significantly reduce fractures it is helpful to know that in medicine the word "significant" carries a specific meaning: that *the measured change is unlikely to have occurred by chance*. When a result is "statistically significant," it does not mean that the change or benefit was large, or that the studied population received any noticeable benefit. It just means that the drug has brought about a change that has been demonstrated to be true beyond a reasonable doubt. Thus, if a treatment has been shown to significantly increase bone density, it doesn't mean it will make a difference to the life of the individual who takes it.

Claims that a certain drug will "prevent" fracture really mean that the drug reduces a person's *risk* for fracture by a certain percentage. For example, an advertisement for Fosamax claims that women with low bone density who took Fosamax in clinical tests experienced 44 percent fewer vertebral fractures compared to women receiving a placebo. That sounds impressive, but in reality, the benefit was very small. In the Fracture Intervention Trial, the large Fosamax trial, after three years, 2.1 percent (43 women) taking Fosamax suffered a vertebral fracture, compared with 3.8 percent (78 women) who took the placebo. This was a difference of 35 fractures among 4,134 women. The reduction stated in the advertisement was 44 percent, but it was 44 percent of the already small 3.8 percent fracture rate [1]. The actual reduction in fractures is only 1.7 percent.

When these results were released, many experts concluded that the Fosamax trial showed no real benefit at all. The minimal reduction in fractures — many of which were vertebral fractures detected on X-ray and not necessarily the type of fracture that causes pain or symptoms — did not provide sufficient evidence to treat [2].

What is Your Chance of Preventing Fracture?

One way to examine the effectiveness of a treatment is to consider the numbers needed to treat, or NNT. This medical term refers to the number of patients who must be treated to prevent, in this case, one fracture in one person over a defined number of years. The NNTs tell an interesting story.

For example, Fosamax is also claimed to reduce hip fractures by 50 percent. In a study of 2,027 postmenopausal women with osteoporosis and previous fracture, after three years there were 22 hip fractures in the women who took placebo (2.2 percent), and 11 in the Fosamax group (1.1 percent). The actual reduction was 1 percent, not 50 percent. Based on these statistics *90 women* would need to be treated for three years to prevent one hip fracture. The remaining 89 would receive no benefit [3].

If a woman has low bone density (osteopenia), but no previous fractures, her risk for fracture is low. Any treatment is at best going to marginally reduce an already low risk. It is estimated that up to 270 such women would need to be treated for three years to prevent one vertebral fracture in one of them [4]. When a woman has very low bone density and has had previous fragility fractures (osteoporosis), her risk for fracture is much higher. Even so, it is estimated that 15 women would need to undergo treatment for three years to prevent one vertebral fracture in one of them [5]. It is estimated that literally *hundreds* of women with low bone density or osteopenia would need to be treated more than three years to prevent one hip fracture in one person, if any at all. That means that hundreds would be taking a drug, exposing themselves to side effects, and receiving no benefit [6].

Osteoporosis expert Dr. Ego Seeman of the University of Melbourne, Australia, poses the question: "Should we expose huge numbers of these women [age 50 and with low bone density] to a drug, its costs, inconveniences, side-effects, when most will not sustain a fracture had no treatment been given? That is, most who take the drug will be exposed to the risk of side effects and costs and receive no benefit … This is the nature of preventive medicine; we have to treat large numbers to avert events in few. This is why the drugs we use must be safe — because most exposed do not benefit, and even a small number of adverse events can tip the balance of net benefit to net harm [7]."

Harm vs Benefit

All medications carry side effects and for a drug to be worth taking, the benefits must outweigh the risks. Researchers uncover side effects prior to submitting a drug for approval to the FDA, but just as benefits can be exaggerated, harms that emerge in clinical trials are often played down. And unanticipated side effects can surface long after a drug has been approved. Who hasn't heard the expression, "The cure is worse than the disease"?

Fifty years ago, many in the Western world thought that medicine had discovered the Holy Grail in the form of supplemental estrogen — a hormone treatment claiming to halt the aging process in women, alleviate menopausal symptoms and prevent postmenopausal health risks.

HRT was initially heralded as a health-promoting panacea that would prevent a variety of serious conditions while simultaneously keeping users young. Doctors the world over embraced estrogen replacement (and later combined estrogen with progesterone) while massive marketing campaigns successfully appealed to women's vanity and desire to remain youthful. For many health-conscious women, HRT became the accepted way to manage the ups and downs of the menopause transition — the hot flashes, sweats, sleep disturbances, mood swings, and vaginal dryness — while simultaneously preventing (they were told) heart disease and osteoporosis.

Although justification for use came from trials that were poorly designed or lacked controls, the medical community had become convinced that HRT would prevent age-related heart disease and osteoporosis. Early studies claimed to show a reduced risk for heart disease, the number one killer of women in the United States. And when HRT was found to slow bone density loss through the menopause transition, normal age-related bone loss was identified as a major cause of osteoporosis in older women. Consequently, many women were advised to undergo a long-term HRT regimen to replace the "missing" bone-protective hormones, and to protect their hearts.

The promise that a single pill could prevent age-related chronic diseases was so compelling that millions of healthy women proceeded to take HRT long term for diseases they didn't have and may never have developed. By 2001, hormone replacement therapy was the No. 1 prescription drug *in the world*[8]. By 2002, 38 percent of postmenopausal United States women (some 16 million) were using hormone replacement therapy, making it the most frequently prescribed medication in the United States, accounting for more than $1 billion in sales [9].

Out of the blue, in 2002 the Women's Health Initiative trial (WHI), one of the largest clinical trials of its kind ever undertaken in the United States, was halted prematurely after 5 years when interim results indicated that HRT significantly increased the risk of serious disease.

We now know that combined HRT (estrogen and progesterone) is associated with an increased risk of breast cancer, and death from breast cancer, ovarian cancer, an increased risk for death from lung cancer, stroke, blood clots, and a doubled risk of dementia for women over 65. There is an increased risk for heart attacks when a woman is 70 years or older. Estrogen alone carries an increased risk of stroke, blood clots and dementia. It increases the risk of ovarian cancer after more than five years of use. It may increase the risk of breast cancer. Estrogen alone increases the risk of cancer of the lining of the uterus [10].

The FDA revised labels on both estrogen and estrogen-progesterone replacement therapy to carry a "black box" warning noting the increased risks for heart disease, heart attacks, strokes, and breast cancer. This applies to all brands and types of hormones. Despite some evidence for fracture benefit with long-term use, HRT is no longer recommended for the prevention of osteoporosis.

HRT use in the U.S. has dropped by around 50 percent since 2002 and breast cancer incidence is also in decline. Some 30,000 *fewer* women developed breast cancer in the US in 2003 and 2004 – the lowest rate since 1987. Estrogen-receptor positive tumours (those most likely to be affected by HRT use) declined by a massive 14.7 percent [11]. Another study has found the number of myocardial infarctions, or heart attacks have also declined in menopausal women each year [12].

"Why did the medical and research community ever believe that hormone replacement therapy prevented or treated disease?" asked Adriane Fugh-Berman, M.D. and Cynthia Pearson in their 2002 article, "The Over-Selling of Hormone Replacement Therapy. "Not a single controlled trial ever showed that HRT prevented cardiovascular disease, stroke, Alzheimer's disease, or wrinkles, nor that it was an effective treatment for depression or incontinence [13]."

There is a sobering answer. Physicians rely on medical literature to keep abreast of safety profiles. A colleague's name on a peer-reviewed article gives confidence when making prescribing decisions. It has come to light in 2010 that over several years Wyeth pharmaceuticals hired medical ghost-writers to create favourable articles about HRT. They would later add the name of a reputable physician, giving the appearance that they were the writer. Doctors can be forgiven for believing they were reading reputable commentary. But at what cost to their trusting patients [14]?

Hard on the Heels of HRT: Bisphosphonates and More...

Although initially heralded as safe and effective, serious unpredicted side-effects are emerging for the biphosphonates Fosamax, Actonel, Boniva and Reclast. A lengthening list of side-effects including spontaneous fractures of the thigh bone, osteonecrosis of the jaw, chronic and acute joint bone and muscle pain, inflammatory eye disease, delayed bone healing, and cancer of the esophagus raises serious questions about the widespread prescribing of treatments that do not benefit the majority who take them. In an about-face, the same osteoporosis doctors who for years exhorted women to take bisphosphonates for the rest of their lives and argued fiercely for the drug's safety are now recommending a "drug holiday" after 5 years citing "some anxieties with long-term use [15]."

In place of the bisphosphonates come new drugs: Prolia, that profoundly suppresses bone remodeling and adversely influences the immune system; and Forteo, a drug that appears to rebuild bone but is linked to bone cancer in rats. (See Chapter 6 for more detail).

Drugs for osteoporosis return large fortunes to the pharmaceutical companies that manufacture and patent them. Merck, the manufacturer of Fosamax made 3.2 billion from 22 million Fosamax prescriptions in 2006. And from 1999 to 2009, Fosamax and Fosamax Plus D, had worldwide sales of more than $23.8 billion, according to IMS Health, a health information company that tracks drug sales [16] [17]. Prolia, approved for use by the FDA in June 2010 is predicted to make $2.1 billion for its manufacturer Amgen in 2012 alone [18].

Making an Informed Choice

Ten million people in the United States have been diagnosed with osteoporosis, and health officials estimate that at least 33 million more men and women have undiagnosed low bone density and are at increased risk for osteoporosis. Health officials are urging doctors to identify at-risk patients and proceed with "bone sparing" treatments.

Making the decision to embark on osteoporosis treatment is complex and difficult. The information that follows on current therapy options needs to be viewed in the light of the previous points made in Chapters 1 – 4. Namely, low bone density is not a disease requiring treatment, and a genuine diagnosis of established osteoporosis (bone fracture) is often linked to other factors that should be addressed before considering treatment. Many of these factors involve lifestyle choices that can help create healthy bone and are discussed in Chapter 10. Ultimately, the decision to undergo treatment must involve a careful weighing of the risk for fracture against the risk of embarking on a treatment with serious short and long-term side effects that cannot guarantee prevention of fracture.

***

Chapter 6
The Myth of Safety

Myth #4: Osteoporosis can be safely treated and prevented with drugs.

When examining current osteoporosis treatments, a paradox emerges. Although they may increase bone density, and although they can decrease fracture risk among osteoporotic patients, they do not benefit the majority of people taking them and may actually worsen a patient's condition.

Most of the current treatments do not build new bone or stimulate the growth of new bone. Treatments aim to slow bone density loss and in some cases increase bone density, yet no conclusive evidence exists that these drugs will prevent fractures in an individual with low bone density (osteopenia). Neither is there evidence that they will rebuild fragile bone. The widespread prescribing of medication based on a bone density diagnosis alone has the 'worried well' taking osteoporosis drugs in droves believing they are preventing a disease may never have.

Bone density reveals little about the microstructure and strength of bones. Drugs that can increase bone density are not able to reverse the loss of bone strength that occurs in the type of osteoporosis where the trabecular struts are severed; no bone medication has been shown to rebuild severed connections. Thus, a treatment that significantly increases bone density will not necessarily reduce fracture rates, alleviate pain, or prevent disability.

Bisphosphonates

Bisphosphonates, the most widely prescribed of all osteoporosis drugs, are synthetic compounds that bind to bone mineral crystals and inhibit bone resorption. They are known to be effective in slowing bone loss and can increase bone density in the short term. The action of bisphosphonates is not fully understood. What is known is that they effectively poison and kill bone-remodelling cells, and in the process disrupt the underlying physiology of bone metabolism.

Bisphosphonates are unusually long-acting medications. Their half-life (continuing effect in the body) is estimated to exceed 10 years and the amount of drug within the bone will accumulate with use. Stopping usage means that exposure to the drug continues indefinitely for better or worse. There is no known method of removing the medication from the bones.

One hundred and fifty years ago bisphosphonates were used for making soap and de-scaling boilers. In humans they permanently adhere to the surface of bone, particularly on sites where there is active bone turnover. The cells that reabsorb old or damaged bone (osteoclasts) quite literally swallow a dose of the drug when resorbing the bone. Once inside the osteoclast cell the bisphosphonate poisons a key enzyme, which switches off the cell's ability to function and causes it to die.

For a time the cells that rebuild bone (osteoblasts) will continue to function – hence the increase in bone density observed with the use of the drugs – but they eventually die as well, as they require the action of osteoclast cells to stimulate their action. Thus although bisphosphonates may favourably influence bone density loss, their mechanism of action suppresses the bone remodelling process.

As early as 2000 concerns were raised that long-term use might produce an older skeleton of more crystallized bone with less tensile strength in places like the hip [1]. Osteoporosis authority Dr. Ego Seeman cautioned that "over time, this process may produce a thinned and brittle structure that may be prone to structural failure [2]." And in 2005, Dr Susan Ott, Associate Professor of Medicine at the University of Washington warned: "The bisphosphonates in doses used today suppress bone formation to a greater extent than the other antiresorbing medications, so it is possible that microdamage accumulation would develop after 15 or 20 yr—just about the time between menopause and the usual onset of osteoporotic fractures. Certainly this is an issue that requires long-term, carefully designed research [3]."

These concerns did nothing to stem the avalanche of bisphosphonate prescriptions for millions of users worldwide. But in 2010 accumulating cases of catastrophic osteonecrosis (bone death) of the jaw, delayed healing, and increasing evidence for spontaneous fractures of the femur in women who have used the drugs for 5 or more years, may be proving these few early voices right. These drugs may be causing the very problem they are supposed to prevent.

Oral bisphosphonate administration can be difficult. The drugs must be taken on an empty stomach to prevent potentially serious stomach problems and to maximize absorption. Food must be avoided for up to two hours. It is necessary to remain upright for at least 30 minutes because of the risk of irritating or even making holes in the wall of the esophagus. Daily regimens have now been replaced by weekly or monthly doses and some bisphosphonates are administered once-yearly by injection. These unpleasant effects may explain why almost 50 percent of patients prescribed oral osteoporosis drugs reportedly discontinue their treatment within six months [4].)

Bisphosphonates should not be used by younger women of child-bearing years. Dr Susan Ott, Associate Professor of Medicine at the University of Washington warns: "Studies in animals show fetal and maternal abnormalities in bones and calcium metabolism, so it is unethical to study this medication in pregnant women or women who might become pregnant while the bisphosphonate is still in the bones [5]."

Bisphosphonate Brands

Bisphosphonates are relatively new drugs. Merck's Fosamax was first used in the 1990s and other versions have followed. Fosamax (alendronate) Actonel (risedronate) and Boniva (ibandronate) are oral bisphosphonates currently approved by the FDA for the treatment of osteoporosis in both women and men. They are also indicated for the treatment of Paget's disease, hypercalcemia, skeletal metastatic disease, and other bone diseases. Atelvia is a delayed-release formulation of the currently marketed product Actonel. It is FDA approved for the prevention and treatment of postmenopausal osteoporosis and glucocorticoid-induced osteoporosis, for men with osteoporosis, and the treatment of Paget's disease of bone.

First approved by FDA in 1995 Fosamax is the most widely prescribed oral bisphosphonate used by more than 20 million people worldwide. It ranks as the 21st most prescribed drug on the market. The drug generated worldwide sales for manufacturer Merck of more than $23.8 billion from 1999 to 2009 before its patent expired in 2008 [6].

The intravenous bisphosphonates are Reclast, Zometa Zomera, Aclasta (all brand names for zoledronic acid) and Aredia (pamidronate). In 2007 the FDA approved a single 5mg infusion of Reclast for the treatment and prevention of postmenopausal osteoporosis. It is also approved for the treatment of osteoporosis in men, the treatment and prevention of glucocorticoid-induced osteoporosis, and treatment of Paget's disease of bone Zometa is approved for the treatment of hypercalcemia, of malignancy and multiple myeloma and bone metastases.

Pamidronate's efficacy in reducing fracture has not been established. Acute and delayed hypersensitivity reactions can occur with intravenous pamidronate, and its use is contraindicated in patients with vitamin D deficiency, since the drug can cause a precipitous drop in serum calcium levels.

Etidronate (Didronel) and **clodronate (Bonefos)** were the first bisphosphonates. Neither drug is approved in the US for the treatment of osteoporosis. Etidronate is approved for use in New Zealand and Canada. Bonefos is used in some cancers to reduce bone destruction that could result in bone pain and fractures. It is also used to bring down high calcium blood levels to normal as well as maintain normal calcium blood levels.

Benefits of Bisphosphonates

Bisphosphonates like Fosamax are prescribed to prevent hip, wrist or vertebral fracture. Yet overall their fracture benefit is minimal. Primary osteoporosis prevention applies to those who have DXA T-scores greater than -2.5 (osteopenia) and have not had a previous osteoporotic or fragility fracture. Bisphosphonates are not recommended for primary prevention as the evidence shows no fracture benefit [7].

Secondary osteoporosis prevention applies to those who have T-scores less than -2.5 (osteoporosis) along with existing osteoporotic fractures. For people in this category studies have found some vertebral fracture benefit with Fosmax, Actonel and Boniva. But even then the drug will not benefit the majority who take it. Twenty two older women would need to take Fosamax for three years to prevent one vertebral fracture discernible by X-ray in one of them and 90 women would need to be treated for three years to prevent one hip fracture in one of them [8].

Summary of Fracture Benefit

The Cochrane Collaboration provides non-biased authoritative interpretations of medical evidence. Following a review of eleven randomized controlled Fosamax trials published between 1966 to 2007 representing 12,068 women, Cochrane reviewers estimated the following:

1. For higher risk women that have osteoporosis or have already had a vertebral fracture:

- 12 out of 100 women had a vertebral fracture when taking a placebo,

and six out of 100 women had a vertebral fracture when taking Fosamax.

- Two out of 100 women had a fracture in the hip or wrist when taking a placebo, and one out of 100 women had a fracture in the hip or wrist when taking Fosamax.

2. For lower risk women whose bone density is closer to normal [osteopenia] or who have not previously fractured:

- Three out of 100 women had a vertebral fracture when taking a placebo and 1 out of 100 women had a vertebral fracture when taking Fosamax.

- One out of 100 women had a hip fracture when taking a placebo and 1 out of 100 women had a hip fracture when taking Fosamax;
- Three out of 100 women had a wrist fracture when taking a placebo and 4 out of 100 women had a wrist fracture when taking Fosamax;
- 13 out of 100 women had a fracture somewhere other than the spine when taking a placebo, and 12 out of 100 women had a fracture somewhere other than the spine when taking Fosamax [9].

Longer use is not necessarily better. An extended major study found that, over a ten-year period, women who took Fosamax for five years had the same fracture risk as those who took it for ten years [10]. Oral bisphosphonates are no longer recommended for more than five years.

Actonel

The benefits of Actonel are similar to those found with Fosamax. Two separate placebo-controlled studies have found that Actonel increases bone mineral density and reduces the incidence of vertebral fractures in women who have had previous vertebral fractures [11] [12]. A study of postmenopausal women with low bone density but no previous fractures found that three years of Actonel reduced the risk of first vertebral fracture. The researchers advise that 15 such women would need to be treated for three years to prevent one such fracture [13]. However, a study measuring the effect of Actonel on hip fracture in 5,445 elderly women found small benefit only. After three years of use, women less than 80 years old with osteoporosis had a 1.9 percent incidence of hip fracture compared with 3.2 percent of the placebo group [14]. In other words, if 100 women took the drug for three years, it would save just over one hip fracture.

Boniva

Despite its more convenient monthly dosage, and despite being vigorously promoted by actress Sally Field, Boniva's benefits lag behind those of Fosmax and

Actonel. From randomized clinical trial evidence the three drugs should offer equivalent effect, but in 2010 the US health insurer WellPoint conducted internal research on 26,000 of its members which linked Boniva to higher fracture rates, lower patient compliance and higher total costs of care than Fosamax and Actonel [15].

Zolendronic acid (Reclast)

Reclast was approved by the FDA in 2007 for the prevention and treatment of osteoporosis. In a 3-year trial of 7765 postmenopausal women with osteoporosis an annual Reclast injection reduced vertebral and hip fracture incidence [16]. Recent studies indicate that an annual dose of zoledronic acid may also prevent recurring fractures in patients with a previous hip fracture [17].

A further study has shown that bone turnover remains suppressed in postmenopausal women for up to three years from a single 5mg injected dose. It is not known whether such a dosing interval reduces fracture [18].

Although an annual injected dose is seen to be an easier option than oral bisphosphonates, if a patient experiences an adverse event there is nothing to be done. There is no antidote, the drug cannot be removed from the body. Side effects discussed below can range from osteonecrosis of the jaw to joint bone and muscle pain, atrial fibrillation, flu-like symptoms and the potential for spontaneous fracture.

Side Effects of Bisphosphonates
Atrial fibrillation

Atrial fibrillation is an abnormal heart rhythm that reduces cardiac output and increases stroke risk. Overall mortality rates are doubled in patients with atrial fibrillation.

A large study found atrial fibrillation to be nearly three times more common among women taking Zoledronate or Reclast. Of 3,889 women using the drug and 3,876 given placebo injections, one in 77 Reclast patients developed the problem [19].

And in the large FIT study involving 6,459 women, half of whom took Fosamax while half took a placebo, 47 of the women taking Fosamax developed atrial fibrillation, compared to 31 cases in the placebo group [20].

However a 2008 FDA review based on information provided by the manufacturers concluded that the risk was minimal. "After our review, based on the data available at this time, healthcare professionals should not alter their prescribing patterns for bisphosphonates and patients should not stop taking their bisphosphonate medication [21]."

But the authors of a 2009 meta-analysis of randomized controlled trials advised that the atrial fibrillation risk should not be dismissed, and that clinicians should increase the monitoring of their patients [22].

Osteonecrosis of the Jaw

A painful condition that is difficult to treat, osteonecrosis (bone death) of the jaw is defined as the presence of exposed bone in the mouth, which fails to heal after appropriate intervention. Cases associated with bisphosphonate use were first reported in 2004 following either simple tooth extraction or denture trauma that resulted in jawbone exposure [23]. Bisphosphonates appear to make bacterial infection of the mouth and jaw tissue more aggressive and of a type that is resistant to many antibiotic treatments [24].

There is presently no known prevention for bisphosphonate-associated osteonecrosis of the jaw (BONJ). Treatment includes stopping bisphosphonate therapy for more than 6 months, long-term antibiotics, and various surgical procedures.

The majority of cases of jawbone necrosis come after someone has been treated for cancer with potent, intravenous forms of the drugs such as Zometa or Reclast, and pamidronate (Aredia). About 1 in 5 cancer patients treated with these bisphosphonates develop the problem and studies have estimated that BONJ occurs in 0-0.04 percent of patients taking orally administered bisphosphonates [25].

However, a study conducted at the University of Southern California School of Dentistry, found that 4 percent of dental patients taking Fosamax had osteonecrosis of the jaw. All were women of average age 73 who had been taking the drug for 12 months or longer. Investigator Parish P. Sedghizadeh and colleagues say their findings contradict Fosamax manufacturer's claims that jaw osteonecrosis is a rare side effect of its drug. "We have been told that the risk with oral bisphosphonates is negligible, but 4 percent is not negligible [26]."

The problem may be both total dose absorbed, and total length of exposure. Even though the oral bisphosphonate dose is lower than intravenous forms, long-term use of Fosamax and Actonel means the drug accumulates in the body. Given the large numbers taking bisphosphonates, as longer-term use (more than 10 or 15 years) occurs, the prevalence of BONJ could increase dramatically.

Merck currently faces about 1,000 Fosamax lawsuits over their failure to adequately warn consumers and the medical community about the risk of osteonecrosis of the jaw, which prevented many doctors from taking preventative actions that could have reduced the risk of aggravating the Fosamax dental injury. The first lawsuits were filed in about 2006 [27].

Cancer of the Esophagus

People who take bisphosphonates for several years may have an increased risk of esophageal cancer. In 2008 in a letter to the New England Journal of Medicine, Diane Wysowski, an epidemiologist at the FDA, reported that since the initial marketing of Fosamax in 1995, the FDA had received 23 reports in which patients developed esophageal tumors. Typically, two years lapsed between the start of the drug and the development of esophageal cancer [28].

Although uncommon, and although studies have brought conflicting results, a recent study from the UK found that after about five years' use of the drug, the risk for people aged 60 to 79 was doubled from 1 in 1000 to 2 in 1000 [29].

In a 2010 editorial in the BMJ, FDA epidemiologist Diane Wysowski, noted the FDA has collected a total of 68 case reports of esophageal cancer in patients taking bisphosphonates - half in the United States and the rest in Europe and Japan. The FDA has not ordered label warnings regarding this possible risk [30].

Bisphosphonates can cause inflammation in the esophagus that could make cancer more likely. "The possibility of adverse effects on the esophagus should prompt doctors who prescribe these drugs to consider risks versus benefits," wrote Diane Wysowski. She also said patients should take the medicines carefully, with a full glass of water before eating and not reclining for at least 30 minutes afterward.

Joint bone and muscle pain

Hundreds of women and men using Fosamax and Actonel report on patient websites such as askapatient.com that they are experiencing chronic, often severe, joint and bone pain, swelling of ankles and feet, muscles cramping and stiffness, and difficulty walking, sometimes after just one dose of the drug. A 2005

Serious Adverse Events report from the U.S. Food and Drug Administration describes Fosamax-related bone joint and muscle pain as 'severe,' 'extreme,' 'disabling,' or 'incapacitating.' "Many patients were unable to walk, climb stairs, or perform usual activities. Some became bedridden, and others required walkers, crutches, or wheelchairs." They caution that "underreporting of pain is probably considerable because of its subjective nature and because physicians may attribute pain to osteoporosis [31]."

Spontaneous Fractures of the Femur

There have long been concerns that the bisphosphonate action of suppressing bone turnover may cause bone to deteriorate in strength and become more brittle over time. Recent medical literature has been inundated with reports and studies linking bisphosphonate drugs to atypical spontaneous mid-femur (thigh bone) fractures.

In October 2010 the FDA issued a press release warning of possible risk of femur fractures caused by the Fosamax, Boniva, Actonel and Reclast or Zometa, and ordered this warning to appear on the drug labelling. An American Society of Bone and Mineral Research (ASBMR) task force had found 310 cases of spontaneous fracture of the femur in which 94 percent of patients were taking bisphosphonates [32].

Reports of these unexpected and disturbing events began to surface in 2005 from the US, then Singapore, Australia, Sweden and Hong Kong [33][34][35][36]. All have a similar story to tell: the thighbones of women patients on Fosamax for five years or more have simply snapped while they were walking or standing. Some individuals experienced hip and thigh pain leading up to the event, and others had no warning. Biopsies after fracture have shown severely depressed bone formation. These fractures don't appear to heal well even with the best of treatment. A physician describing her own experience noted that healing was so slow she couldn't resume normal activity for two years [37].

That fractures are occurring in these numbers indicates a possible epidemic, as only a small percentage of adverse effects are ever reported. Busy doctors may not take the time to report, and hospital records are not readily accessed. The ASMBR report of October 2010 cautions, "There is concern that lack of awareness and underreporting may mask the true incidence of the problem [38]." To date almost all reports in the medical literature involve Fosamax the oldest and most widely used bisphosphonate. The newer the bisphosphonate, the fewer number of fractures reported, but that may be because it takes time for reports to surface.

Women who sustain these fractures are often told they are due to the underlying osteoporosis, not the drug. But Dr. Felicia Cosman, clinical director of the National Osteoporosis Foundation notes in a November 2010 LA Times article "It's ironic that many of these cases of femur factures were in women with mild bone loss who probably should not have been on these drugs…We probably used too many bisphosphonates in too many women for too many years [39]."

Osteoporosis authority Dr Susan Ott had warned in 2005 that long-term suppression of bone remodelling might lead to fracture [40]. In a July 2008 New York Times article she admitted to having seen instances of spontaneous fracture: "I have several similar patients myself. ... Prior to these recent articles, there were a few cases here and a few cases there, but they are kind of starting to add up [41]." In October 2010 at the 2010 ASBMR meeting in Toronto Susan Ott presented more cases. Over a three-year period, Californian Kaiser Permanente doctors reported 135 atypical femur fractures out of a total of 16,000 broken femurs. Almost all (96.4 percent) of the 135 individuals were on bisphosphonates and the rate of atypical fractures appeared to rise with longer duration of use. Dr Ott reported these atypical fractures have a characteristic X-ray appearance. The fracture line is straight through the mid-shaft of the bone, and the outer margin thickened, suggesting stress fracture as a result of microfracture. Patients typically report pain in the area for weeks or months before the actual fracture [42]. It has also been observed that when a fracture has occurred in one leg, a second atypical fracture may occur in the other thigh [43].

A team of physicians and epidemiologists in Toronto assessed the treatment and fracture data of 205,466 women in Ontario aged 68 or older who had been treated with bisphosphonates. They identified 716 women who sustained a fracture of the femur or thigh after starting bisphosphonate treatment. They also found that those who had taken the drugs for five years or longer were more than twice as likely to have had a thigh bone fracture as those who took them only briefly [44].

New recommendations are to take a drug 'holiday' if you have been taking bisphosphonates for more than five years and to consider alternative osteoporosis medication. But replacing bisphosphonates with an alternative new drug may not necessarily be better. These drugs can also drastically interfere with bone metabolism, and long-term effects are yet to be revealed.

Other Treatments

Prolia (denosumab)

Pioneered by the biotechnology company Amgen, genetically engineered Prolia is the newest approved bone treatment. Despite concerns raised by FDA staff in 2009 that the new treatment may bring serious risks, the FDA approved its use in June 2010 for postmenopausal women with osteoporosis who are at high risk for fractures; or those who are intolerant to other osteoporosis therapies. It is also approved for use in men [45].

It is heralded as more effective and easier to use than the oral bisphosphonates as it is administered by injection 6 monthly, doesn't accumulate in the body and has no known esophageal side effects. It will cost around US$1,650 per year, making it a competitive alternative to other osteoporosis treatments. Sales in the three months following its FDA approval reached $10 million [46]. The revenue projection for 2012 is $2.1 billion [47].

In a three year clinical trial (funded by Amgen) of 7,868 postmenopausal women with osteoporosis, there was a 4.8 percent absolute risk reduction of vertebral fractures (264 in the placebo group and 86 in the Prolia group), a 0.3 percent absolute risk reduction of hip fractures (47 in placebo group and 27 in the drug group) and a 1.5 percent absolute risk reduction of non-vertebral (hip wrist and rib) fractures (316 with placebo vs 253 with Prolia). Prolia was also found to significantly increase bone density in that period [48].

Just how the precise orchestration of the body's constant bone remodelling works is still far from understood, but Amgen's research identified the protein RANK Ligand (RANKL), a molecule that appears to activate osteoclast function in the bone resorption process, as well as playing a vital role in the body's defences against infection. It then created Prolia, a genetically engineered human monoclonal antibody that mimics osteoprotegerin, a tumor necrosis factor cytokine that naturally binds to and inhibits RANKL. (Cytokines are chemical messengers that help regulate the nature and intensity of an immune response.) In mimicking osteoprotegerin, Prolia deactivates RANKL, preventing osteoclasts from reabsorbing or breaking down bone. This allows osteoblasts to rebuild bone unopposed for a time (which explains the increase in bone density) until they too cease to exist and bone remodelling is fully suppressed.

It is likely that adverse effects won't show up for some time. Like HRT and the bisphosphonates that have gone before, Prolia goes onto the market with no long term testing. A 2009 FDA review cautioned that Prolia may produce unhealthy changes in bone structure. It warned that because of the marked suppression of bone turnover, the drug is likely to cause osteonecrosis of the jaw, spontaneous atypical fractures, and delayed healing as bisphosphonates have. A few cases of jawbone necrosis have already been reported.

In addition, there is a risk of infections and cancers. FDA staff expressed concerns that Prolia could promote cancerous tumor development. When they pooled data from all the postmenopausal osteoporosis trials with Prolia, the results suggested "a slightly increased incidence" of breast, pancreatic, gastrointestinal, and reproductive-tract tumors. They observed twice as many women discontinued Prolia versus placebo during the trials because of breast cancer [49].

Other side effects include skin infections, predominantly cellulitis, some serious enough to require hospitalization, and other infections such as in the ears, urinary tract, upper respiratory tract and the heart. Sciatica, cataracts, constipation, rash, excema, hypocalcaemia (low calcium levels in the blood, pain in extremity, back pain and pain in the muscles and bones, and elevated cholesterol levels have also been reported.

Evista (Raloxifene)

Evista, is one of a drug class known as selective estrogen receptor modulators or SERMS. SERMS are anti-estrogenic — that is, they work differently from estrogen in that they don't appear to cause an increase of cancer cells in the breast, but still have an antiresorptive effect on bone.

As often happens in medicine, a drug prescribed for a certain purpose will show risks and benefits in unexpected ways.

Tamoxifen is also a SERM and is prescribed for women who have had breast cancer. In the late 1980s, researchers noted that women taking tamoxifen had increased bone density.

Since then, Evista has been developed as a treatment specifically for osteoporosis. It has been approved by the FDA for prevention of postmenopausal bone loss. In September 2007, the U.S. Food and Drug Administration approved using Evista to reduce the risk of breast cancer in post-menopausal women at high risk. Evista is also approved to reduce breast cancer risk in post-menopausal women with osteoporosis [50].

In Evista trials that lasted up to eight years —breast cancer was diagnosed in 2.5 percent of the women taking a placebo and one percent of the women taking Evista. It is not clear whether the drug prevents breast cancer or simply delays its onset [51].

The Multiple Outcomes of Raloxifene Evaluation (MORE) study involving 7,705 postmenopausal women is one of the largest osteoporosis trial ever conducted.

The participants averaged 70 years of age and had all been diagnosed with osteoporosis. Evista increased bone density by 3 percent and reduced vertebral fractures by about 40 percent after three to four years. In other words, 22 women with osteoporosis would need to be treated for four years to prevent one of them having a vertebral fracture. In the group with low bone density and previous vertebral fracture, the number needed to treat is 12 [52]. There is no evidence that Evista will prevent hip fracture.

Evista can increase menopausal symptoms of hot flashes and leg cramps swelling of the legs and feet, flu-like symptoms, joint pain, and sweating, and also poses a threefold-increased risk for blood clots in the legs and lungs and death due to stroke. The FDA advises that women with current or prior blood clots in the legs, lungs, or eyes should not take Evista [53].

Unlike tamoxifen, Evista does not appear to stimulate the lining of the uterus, and is therefore less likely to be associated with an increased risk of cancer of the uterus.

More SERMS are in the pipeline. In a five year trial of 8556 postmenopausal women with osteoporosis, at a dose of 0.5 mg per day, lasofoxifene was associated with reduced risks of non-vertebral and vertebral fractures, estrogen-receptor positive breast cancer, coronary heart disease, and stroke, but an increased risk of blood clots in the lungs and leg cramps [54]. It is unapproved for use at the time of writing (January 2011).

Forteo (Teriparatide)

In 2002, the FDA approved teriparatide (Forteo) a genetically engineered form of human parathyroid hormone, for people with severe osteoporosis and vertebral compression fractures; those who have fractures despite prolonged bisphosphonate use; those with a very high risk of fractures and low bone formation, and those patients with osteoporosis as a result of prolonged use of high dose prednisone.

An anabolic treatment, the action of Forteo increases the formation of new bone whereas other osteoporosis drugs block the resorption of bone. Like naturally produced parathyroid hormone it stimulates osteoblasts, increasing their bone building activity. Patients are required to give themselves daily injections using needles, much like those used by diabetics.

Forteo appears to significantly reduce vertebral and non-vertebral fractures. A trial of 1637 postmenopausal women with prior vertebral fractures who received Forteo or placebo found that 14 percent of the women taking placebo had new vertebral fractures, and 5 percent of the women taking Forteo had vertebral fractures after about 19 months. There were also a statistically significant lower number of non-vertebral fractures in the Forteo treated group. Forteo increased spine and hipbone density [53].

When Forteo was administered for 12 weeks to 145 patients that had painful non-healing pelvic fractures that persisted for 6 months or longer, 93 percent of the group showed significant healing and almost complete elimination of pain in what was reported as half the time it would normally take [56].

And in an ironic twist, two new articles in 2010 suggest that Forteo may combat osteonecrosis of the jaw (ONJ) and other fractures caused by bisphosphonates. One article details the collected data on how Forteo has been seen to stimulate bone growth in patients suffering ONJ. The other article details how Forteo was used specifically to reverse the effects of ONJ from Fosamax in an 88-year-old woman in a matter of weeks [57].

Forteo comes with a "black box" warning on the packaging. When rats were injected with high doses of the medication, they developed a rare bone cancer. For this reason, treatment is currently not recommended for more than two years. The effects of this drug go away very quickly, so consumers are often advised to follow it with bisphosphonate or other therapy.

Forteo is not indicated for children and adolescents, those who have had radiation therapy, those with Paget's disease, hypercalcemia or hyperparathyroidism, gout or high uric acid and women who are pregnant or nursing. There is also concern that the increase in bone turnover and associated increase in bone porosity with Forteo use may offset some of the apparent positive effects on bone strength [58].

In trials, Forteo was associated with a slight increase in dizziness, leg cramps, headache, and nausea.

The cost of teriparatide is several-fold higher than that of other therapies.

Vitamin D

Recent studies suggest that vitamin D deficiency is affecting at least one billion people worldwide [59]. Severe vitamin D deficiency is prevalent among people who avoid the sun or have darker skin, have diabetes or kidney disease, and among many elderly or unwell people who may be institutionalized or confined indoors [60]. With many people covering the skin to avoid sunburn and skin cancer, the prevalence of vitamin D depletion in adults is believed to be increasing. A study of veiled Muslim women living in Denmark found the women needed to supplement with at least three times the recommended daily amount of the vitamin to secure a normal level of vitamin D [61].

Vitamin D deficiency has been found to be as high as 86 percent among older women in rest homes and present in up to 76 percent of women with osteoporosis and 50 - 70 percent of women with a history of fracture [62]. Vitamin D insufficiency has been linked to muscle weakness and pain. Restoring normal levels has been shown to increase muscle strength and reduce falls [63].

A healthy person utilizes approximately 3,000-4,000 IU of vitamin D daily. Vitamin D levels are influenced by age, skin color (fair skin being more absorbent than dark skin), geographical location in terms of proximity to the equator, and how much time is spent outdoors in the sun. A young white person needs approximately four minutes of direct exposure to sunlight on the arms and legs to generate approximately 1000 IU of vitamin D3. Studies show that bathing suit exposure during summer, until skin just begins to turn pink, results in skin production of 10,000-50,000 IU of vitamin D [64]. It is virtually impossible to achieve vitamin D toxicity through sun exposure because within about 20 minutes of ultraviolet exposure in light-skinned individuals (or 3 to 6 times longer for darker-skinned people), concentrations of vitamin D produced in the skin reach equilibrium. After the age of 70, the skin does not convert vitamin D as effectively so older adults will probably not generate sufficient vitamin D naturally from sunlight [65].

There are a few foods that are naturally rich in vitamin D, mainly fatty fish such as salmon, mackerel, and sardines, and fish liver oil. Milk in the US is fortified with 400 IU of vitamin D per quart, as are some cereals, breads, and orange juice.

Other than sun or ultraviolet light exposure the recommended way to ensure adequate vitamin D levels is to use oral dosing of vitamin D3 either daily or intermittently. Vitamin D3 is the preferred supplement for adults. Vitamin D2 is not recommended for routine supplementation. It is advisable to have vitamin D levels in the blood tested before embarking on treatment and then again after 3-4 months. The Serum 25-Hydroxyvitamin D or 25(OH)D blood test indicates the supply of vitamin D available in the body. (The test doesn't reveal the amount of vitamin D stored in other body tissues; it's not so easy to test for that.)

Optimum levels of vitamin D are hotly debated. Renowned researcher Dr Robert Heaney has demonstrated that calcium absorption is 65 percent higher when blood vitamin D levels average 34 ng/m (86nmol/L) compared to 20 ng/mL (50nmol/L) [66]. Controversially, a 2010 report from the US Institute of Medicine (IOM) has determined that almost all people are sufficient with a blood 25(OH)D level of 20 ng/mL (50 nmol/L). With a few exceptions, the IOM does not recommend vitamin D supplementation. However it does recommend a daily intake of 800IU for adults over the age of 70 years, and 600IU for adults aged 51-70 with a maximum daily intake of 4000IU [67]. But guidelines from Osteoporosis Canada issued around the same time call for a level between 30-32 ng/ml (75 and 80 nmol/L) [68].

Dr Heaney argues that if a 32 ng/ mL 25(OH)D blood level was to be accepted in the United States as the necessary minimum for preventing bone loss, a minimum daily intake of 2,600 IU of vitamin D3 would meet the needs of 97 percent of U.S. residents [69]. Similarly osteoporosis researcher Bischoff-Ferrari estimates 700-1,000 IU vitamin D supplementation for eight weeks will result in less than half of average healthy adults achieving serum vitamin D levels of 30 ng/mL [70]. Dr Heaney advises that the safe upper intake level for vitamin D3 is 10,000IU. Blood levels of 25(OH)D can be expected to rise by about 1 ng/mL (2.5 nmol/L) for every 100 IU of additional vitamin D each day.

Higher doses appear to offer protection from fracture. A meta-analysis demonstrated that a daily dose of 400 IU was not effective for fracture prevention but that doses of vitamin D at 700-800 IU daily reduced the risk for hip fracture by 26 percent and any non-vertebral fracture by 23 percent compared with either calcium supplements or placebo [71]. A further large meta-analysis, published in 2007, included 29 randomized controlled trials of a total of 63,897 men and women over age 50 and found that calcium and vitamin D in combination was found to be associated with a reduction of any fractures. This reduction in risk was greatest among elderly people who were most regular with the therapy and among those who received at least 1200mg of calcium and 800 IU of vitamin D daily. The number of people needed to treat to prevent one fracture was 53 [72].

It is argued that sufficient levels of vitamin D can lower the required level of calcium intake and it may be that vitamin D supplementation alone is adequate when combined with a diet that covers calcium needs.

In her evaluation of the evidence, osteoporosis authority Dr Susan Brown maintains "Vitamin D serum sufficiency levels [a minimum of 32 ng/mL] could provide for a 50- to 60-percent fracture reduction. …Providing for vitamin D sufficiency is the simplest, most life-supporting, and most cost-effective means of significantly reducing the incidence of osteoporotic fractures worldwide [73]."

Calcitonin

Calcitonin is a natural hormone found in our bodies. It is made by the thyroid gland

and controls the activity of osteoclasts, the cells that reabsorb bone. Calcitonin is also found in certain fish, including salmon, and has been extracted for use as a drug to treat the bone disease known as Paget's disease, and also osteoporosis. Salmon calcitonin was first approved for the treatment of osteoporosis in 1984 in the United States. It appears to have few risks associated with use.

Although previously administered by injection, a nasal spray form of calcitonin has been approved for the treatment of osteoporosis in women who are five years post menopause. A placebo-controlled trial of 1,255 postmenopausal women with low bone density and one or more previous vertebral fractures found that calcitonin treatment slowed bone density loss and reduced new vertebral fractures over a five-year period. There is no evidence of hip fracture prevention [74]. Calcitonin has been found to have analgesic qualities in the management of severe pain due to vertebral crush fractures [75].

When osteoporosis has occurred as a result of treatment from corticosteroids, calcitonin may be an effective treatment. A study showed that calcitonin appears to preserve bone mass in the first year of glucocorticoid therapy at the lumbar spine by about 3 percent compared to placebo, but not at the femoral neck (hip) [76].

The most common side effects are nasal dryness and irritation, back and joint pain, and headache. It is advised that the drug should be administered with calcium and vitamin D.

Fluoride

There is considerable controversy about the effects of fluoride on bone strength and fracture risk. It is one of the few treatments known to stimulate osteoblast activity and actually increase bone density — an apparently desirable outcome. But increased bone density does not necessarily mean stronger bone. Experience with fluoride has shown that past a certain point, bone may in fact become more brittle and fracture more easily.

In her Web site, Osteoporosis and Bone Physiology, Dr. Susan Ott writes:

In a large well-designed randomized, blinded clinical trial, women who used fluoride for four years had increased fracture rates compared to placebo controls. The bone density of the spine increased by 32 percent, but the hip did not show increased density and the rate of hip fractures was nearly three times as high in the fluoride group. At this time fluoride cannot be recommended for clinical use. Because it is one of the few medications that can enhance osteoblast activity, it thus deserves further research [77].

There is some evidence that fluoridated water is linked to an increased risk of hip fracture, suggesting that even exposure to low levels of fluoride may put elderly people at greater risk [78]. A 1995 study of elderly women in 75 parishes in southwestern France found that the risk of hip fracture was 86 percent greater in those areas with water fluoride concentrations above 0.11 parts per million (ppm) [79]. Optimal concentrations of fluoride in U.S. drinking water are considered to be between 0.7 and 1.2 milligrams per liter (0.11 milligrams per liter (mg/L) is the same as 0.11 parts per million) [80].

Strontium Ranelate (Protelos or Protos)

Natural strontium is a naturally occurring element that is stable and non-radioactive and not to be confused with man-made strontium-90, a radioactive form that is extremely toxic in high doses. Unlike other osteoporosis treatments, strontium appears to decrease bone resorption and stimulate bone formation at the same time.

While little is known about the risks and benefits of strontium nutritional supplements, the patented prescription preparation, strontium ranelate appears to offer some benefit. An independent 2006 Cochrane review of the evidence found that in postmenopausal women who have osteoporosis strontium ranelate increased bone

density and decreased vertebral fractures, but offered little or no benefit in preventing hip or other fractures. Thirteen out of 100 women had spine fractures taking strontium ranelate and 21 out of 100 women had spine fractures taking placebo. One in 3 women had an increase in spine and hip bone mineral density [81].

The Cochrane review also observed that other research indicated risks could include a chance of blood clots and seizures, memory loss and loss of consciousness loss. The cause of these vascular and neurological side effects is not known. Long-term effects of strontium are unknown.

Earlier smaller studies observed decreased bone pain and an increase in bone formation in people taking quite high doses of strontium. These and other independent studies used many different forms of strontium including strontium lactate, gluconate, carbonate, chloride, all of which appear to have a bone building action. Many of these forms have poor gastric tolerance – that is, they are likely to cause upset stomach or diarrhea [82].

Strontium Ranelate is now approved for use in the UK as an alternative to bisphosphonates, but does not have FDA approval in the US.

Progesterone

In recent years, natural progesterone has been popularized for the treatment of menopause symptoms and has been recommended for the prevention of osteoporosis. Natural progesterone is synthesized in a laboratory from the wild yam or from soy. It is what is known as a "bioidentical" hormone, because its molecular structure is identical to the hormone progesterone produced by the ovaries.

There has been some evidence that progesterone enhances the formation of new bone [83]. Progestins (progestagens) used in HRT and contraceptives have been reported to prevent or reverse bone loss in certain clinical situations [84]. But in young women taking injectable medroxyprogesterone acetate (Depo-Provera) for contraception, their bone density was found to be 7 percent lower than young women not using the drug [85].

A randomized controlled trial in the United States, 102 healthy postmenopausal women used progesterone cream and calcium and vitamin supplements. During the one-year study, there was no significant difference in bone density between the progesterone and the control groups [86]. It appears that transdermal natural progesterone, either by itself or in combination with calcium and a multivitamin, has little or no effect on bone mineral density. In the absence of long-term safety data, nature identical hormones must be considered to carry the same risks as conventional HRT.

Ipriflavone

Ipriflavone is a synthetic isoflavone that initially showed promise as an osteoporosis treatment. A randomized controlled trial of 474 postmenopausal women designed to investigate its effectiveness and safety, found little to recommend it [87]. No difference in bone density was seen between the two groups, and in an adverse outcome, some of the women taking ipriflavone had lower levels of certain white blood cells (lymphocytes that are an important part of the immune system) than those taking the placebo.

Summary

While newspaper, magazine, television, and radio advertisements claim effectiveness for the many treatments offered for osteoporosis prevention and treatment, minimal benefit, emerging serious risks, and a lack of evidence from long-term studies should dissuade most people with low bone density from considering these types of treatments. Much of the risk of future fracture can be minimized without having to resort to drug therapy. Many simple, positive steps can be taken to create bone health that will not only benefit the skeleton, but will also benefit overall health and wellbeing.

***

Chapter 7
The Myth of the Magic Bullet

Myth #5: The myth that high calcium intake alone prevents osteoporosis, whether from dairy or supplements.

When it comes to creating bone health through nutrition, one piece of advice seems to drown out all others: "Calcium, particularly from dairy products, builds strong bones." That message is driven home to children and, increasingly, adults — thanks largely to the California Department of Food and Agriculture, which formed the California Milk Processor Board in 1993 to make milk more competitive and increase consumption. Its advertising campaign, franchised nationally since 1995, features celebrities, athletes and movie stars on billboards and in magazines with the famous milk moustache, under the heading, "Got Milk?" The real question, of course, is, "Got Healthy Bones?" — a question of immense concern for everyone wanting to avoid osteoporosis.

Much of the discourse and research concerning nutrition as it relates to bone health, including osteoporosis, has focused on calcium — and with good reason: A mature male skeleton contains more than 1,400 grams of calcium (about 3.1 pounds); a mature female skeleton contains more than 1,200 grams of calcium (about 2.6 pounds). In fact, 99 percent of the body's calcium is found in the bones and teeth. The remaining onepercent of calcium circulates in the blood and has many significant functions. Calcium helps regulate the heartbeat, nervous system, muscle control, enzyme systems, and hormone secretions. Calcium helps cells to cohere and blood to coagulate. If the body lacks enough circulating calcium for these functions, it leaches it from the bones. Even a slight drop in blood calcium levels stimulates the release of calcium from the bones and its absorption from the intestine, at the same time decreasing its loss into the urine. The process is reversed through the actions of vitamin D, parathyroid hormone, and other biochemical agents. In this way bone mineral content is continuously being replenished.

Getting the recommended daily allowance of calcium at all ages is important, preferably from dietary sources. Over the years, however, calcium intake alone has been equated with bone health — another example of the "magic bullet" approach in which a complex condition is solved by a miracle drug or a single nutritional ingredient. In this milieu, many women think that diet has little to do with osteoporosis beyond measuring the calcium levels of foods. However, bone nutritional requirements are much more complex than that, and preventing osteoporosis involves far more than drinking milk on a regular basis. Consider, for example:

* Most women with osteoporosis get plenty of dietary calcium [1].
* Calcium supplementation alone is not proven to build bone [2].
* Countries with the highest rates of osteoporosis are the biggest consumers of dairy products [3].

In reality, bones are complex, dynamic, and alive, and have a wide range of nutritional needs. It is puzzling that the diverse nutritional needs of bone are often ignored, and that those at risk for osteoporosis are regularly advised to supplement with calcium alone. Two of the most important issues that often get overlooked are the body's ability to effectively absorb calcium and how much excess calcium will be excreted from the body — factors which can vary hugely from individual to individual.

An Exquisite Balancing Act

To sustain life, the level of calcium in the blood must be kept within a very narrow range. This is achieved by an exquisitely orchestrated mechanism involving parathyroid hormone and vitamin D, which maintains skeletal calcium and blood calcium in a state of equilibrium.

The body maintains a balance after adjusting for diet, intestinal absorption, excretion, and hormonal functions, as well as growth, physical activity, and disease. For example, research indicates that people excrete between 150 and 250 milligrams of calcium per day — an amount that can fluctuate, depending on factors such as how much protein and sodium a person consumes.

Vitamin D (calcitriol) controls the amount of calcium in the bones. A person who ingests low levels of calcium will have increased levels of circulating calcitriol to improve calcium absorption, whereas a person who receives high levels of calcium will have depressed levels of calcitriol and the calcium will be inefficiently used. People with high-calcium diets excrete more calcium than people with low-calcium intakes, which perhaps explains why osteoporosis is not rampant in countries where people receive low amounts of dietary calcium [4].

Children, Calcium, and Healthy Bones

Many nutrients and mechanisms are involved in the building of peak bone mass in a young person, and even when there is a low calcium intake, a normal peak bone mass can be achieved. Studies of children with low calcium and vitamin D intake in developed and developing countries show that children still achieve a normal peak bone mass despite an apparently deficient diet. The author of a review of the evidence for this phenomenon comments, "It is nearly impossible to explain the robust skeletal mass obtained by so many youngsters who have known nutritional inadequacies of calcium and vitamin D but who are otherwise healthy and active. Nature must somehow be providing well for skeletal growth despite limited intake of the critical nutrient calcium during periods of bone development." He concludes: "The beneficial effect of physical activity may dominate as a determinant of bone mass and bone density early in life [5]."

Increasing Calcium is Not the Answer

Because the amount of calcium in the blood is so carefully regulated, increasing calcium does not necessarily mean that the body will build more bone. Researchers in Madison, Wisconsin, measured the diets and the bone densities of 300 premenopausal women aged 20 to 39, and found that high calcium diets did not result in higher bone density [6]. In fact, too much calcium (more than 2,000 milligrams daily over a long time) can be detrimental. Taken to excess, calcium can cause kidney stones and gallstones.

Calcium supplements (not dietary calcium) may also increase vascular calcification and cardiovascular events. A meta-analysis of nearly 12,000 people enrolled in 11 randomized controlled trials concluded that taking 500mg or more of daily calcium supplementation was associated with a 30 percent increase in the risk of cardiovascular events. The researchers estimated that treating 1000 people with calcium supplements (without additional Vitamin D) for five years would cause an additional 14 heart attacks, 10 strokes, and 13 deaths, and prevent 26 fractures. They caution that "although the magnitude of the increase in risk is modest, the widespread use of calcium supplements means that even a small increase in incidence of cardiovascular disease could translate into a large burden of disease in the population [7]." By contrast, the Women's Health Initiative reported that calcium and vitamin D combined had no effect on the risk of coronary heart disease or stroke [8].

Whether calcium supplementation actually affects bone density and fracture risk is an ongoing debate. Studies have shown both positive and negative results. It would appear that taking calcium, whether as a supplement or via dairy products, seems to have little bone density-increasing effect unless a person's diet is grossly calcium deficient. Most studies have shown that calcium supplementation has little effect on the bone density of the spine, and no effect on the bone density of the hip, the two places where most serious breaks occur [9].

It is generally agreed that calcium intake within the normal dietary range appears to be adequate for bone health. The recommended daily allowance (RDA) for calcium is 1,200 milligrams. High dietary calcium intake has not been shown to lead to stronger bones [10]. Studies of countries with highest rates of hip fracture reveal that they also have the highest dietary intake of calcium — mainly from dairy products [11]. The calcium intake in the Netherlands is high and so is the incidence of osteoporosis [12].

Seriously low calcium intake may lead to deficient bone formation, but this is not borne out by observations of cultures with low calcium intake. A low dietary calcium intake and low BMD have been linked to fewer fractures in Asia and Africa, as well as populations in the United States and Europe [13]. A 1992 review of fracture rates in many countries showed that populations with the lowest calcium intakes had far fewer fractures than those with higher intakes. For example, black South Africans had a very low average calcium intake — only 196 milligrams — yet their fracture incidence was far below that of either black or white Americans [14].

Consider these facts:

- Osteoporosis incidence (as defined by fracture) is highest in those countries where the most (dairy) calcium is consumed: the United States, Australia, New Zealand, Switzerland, the United Kingdom, and Northern Europe [15].

* In The Gambia, the average calcium intake is very low, yet, so is the incidence of osteoporosis (fracture) [16].

Maximizing Calcium Absorption and Minimizing Calcium Loss

Many experts maintain there is no singleuniversal calcium requirement, but rather one that is linked to a person's intake of other nutrients, in particular animal proteins and sodium [17]. Calcium absorption varies enormously from person to person. Clinical trials of postmenopausal women have found that calcium absorption can vary by as much as 61 percent; and that 40 percent of women in calcium balance trials could not absorb enough calcium to stay in balance even with an intake of 800 milligramsper day [18]. A possible explanation is that the women may not have been absorbing adequate levels of calcium due to their high intake of dietary salt or protein [19].

Protein from meat, milk, and eggs contain relatively high concentrations of sulfur amino acids. For every gram of dietary salt consumed, approximately 26 milligrams of calcium is lost in the urine. And for each gram of animal protein consumed, onemilligram of calcium is lost. Thus a 40-gram reduction in animal protein reduces the calcium lost in the urine by 40 milligrams. Assuming that about 20 percent of ingested calcium is absorbed, this lowers a person's daily requirement by 200 milligrams.

Meat-based diets increase the acidity in the blood and urine, as indicated by a lower pH, a measurement indicating the degree of acidity and alkalinity. People who eat meat have an average urine pH of between 4.5 and 5.5, whereas people who do not eat meat have a pH of between 5.5 and 6.5. To buffer the higher acidity and regain equilibrium, the body leaches calcium from the bones. Studies in the United States that compare women who eat meat-based diets with those who eat vegetarian-based diets reach the same conclusion: vegetarian women experience half the bone loss of women who eat meat [20] [22].

The following two studies illustrate the point. Inuit people have a normal to very high intake of dietary calcium — between 500 and 2,500 milligrams per day (mostly from fish bones) — and one of the world's highest intakes of protein — between 250 and 400 grams per day. They also have one of the very highest rates of osteoporosis in the world (as defined by bone mineral density) [23].

African Bantu women, on the other hand, take in only 350 milligrams of calcium per day. Yet, Bantu women never have calcium deficiency, seldom break a bone, and rarely lose a tooth. They consume much less calcium and much less protein than Western populations, and yet are essentially free of osteoporosis. [24]. The Inuit subsist on a meat-based diet consisting of caribou, sea mammals, fish, and birds. The Bantu consume a vegetarian-based diet.

People who have low protein or sodium diets may require lower calcium intakes than those on high protein diets. A 1994 report in the American Journal of Clinical Nutrition showed that when animal proteins were eliminated from the diet, calcium losses were cut in half [25]. The type of food eaten plays a major role in calcium absorption. A study of women in Pittsburgh, Pennsylvania, found that the intake of fat and fiber significantly influences calcium absorption. Surprisingly, women with a higher fat intake and a lower intake of fiber absorbed more calcium. Only certain types of fiber, like wheat bran, seem to reduce calcium absorption. Other forms, such as the fiber found in green, leafy vegetables, including kale, broccoli, and bok choy, did not appear to be detrimental. Women with high blood levels of vitamin D also showed increased absorption, while women with high alcohol intake showed decreased absorption [26].

The role of phosphorus in osteoporosis is unclear, though researchers believe that a dietary ratio of roughly an equal amount of calcium to phosphorus is necessary to maintain normal calcium levels. Because meats contain large amounts of phosphorus, excessive consumption of meat may therefore affect calcium balance.

Phosphates in carbonated drinks can have a similar effect, and there is evidence that teenagers and children who consume carbonated drinks high in phosphoric acid have restricted calcium absorption. Researchers at the Harvard Medical School have found that cola drink consumption increases fracture rates in young girls in the United States [27].

Smoking causes calcium to be lost from the bone and could result in a higher rate of fracture. Researchers studying the bone densities of identical twins found that long-term smokers had a 44 percent greater risk of fracture than their nonsmoking twins [28].

Poor intestinal absorption of calcium may also occur with celiac disease, or gluten intolerance, which remains undetected in many people.

Dairy and Bone

For decades, the dairy industry has convincingly marketed milk as the osteoporosis solution. Most baby boomers and their offspring have been indoctrinated to think that daily milk is a requirement for the growing body and is the ultimate nutrition. Dairy products are said to provide about 70 percent of the dietary calcium of the United States population [29].

It can come as a shock to learn that dairy products could actually contribute to bone loss and fracture. Numerous studies published in journals like the American Journal of Public Health suggest that milk is ineffective in preventing osteoporosis. One study compared milk and calcium consumption in 77,000 women over a 12-year period in relation to the incidence of hip and forearm fractures. It found that those with the highest consumption of dairy products *had more fractures* than those who drank less milk. The authors concluded: "These data do not support the hypothesis that higher consumption of milk and other food sources of calcium by adult women protects against hip or forearm fractures [30]." An Australia study examining the dietary history of elderly residents reached the same conclusion, finding that the consumption of milk and cheese in a person at the age of 20 may be linked to an increased rate of hip fracture when that person becomes at risk in old age [31].

Researchers reviewed 57 studies to determine any correlation between the consumption of dairy foods and bone health. The study found that the majority of outcomes showed no significant relationship between the two. The authors conclude: "The body of scientific evidence appears inadequate to support a recommendation for daily intake of dairy foods to promote bone health in the general U.S. population [32]." And a 2005 analysis of six large prospective trials involving 40,000 men and women found that a low intake of milk was not associated with a significantly increased risk of any fracture – osteoporotic or otherwise [33].

Asia and Osteoporosis

Asian populations have always boasted a much-lower incidence of fragility fracture than Western countries and researchers have linked the rarity of osteoporotic fractures to the traditional Asian diet that is rich in calcium — though not from dairy sources. In 1998, the incidence of hip fracture in MainlandChina was one of the lowest in the world. Although Western food fast food chains and Western foods are gaining popularity, most Asian people still consume a diverse range of fresh vegetables, some fruit, soybeans, fresh seafood, and meats. They typically do not have exposure to refined processed foods, and carbonated drinks, and are not accustomed to eating milk products.

The vast majority of Asian populations are lactose intolerant. The American Journal of Clinical Nutrition estimates that some 80 percent of people in Central Asia, and 90–100 percent in Eastern Asia cannot tolerate dairy consumption [34]. Despite this, the dairy industries of New Zealand, the United States, Europe, and Australia, have aggressively promoted milk consumption to Asian populations in recent years, in particular by targeting the bone health and infant formula markets. Vulnerable mothers abandon breast for bottle believing they are doing best for their child, and older women frightened by the specter of fragility fractures resort to milk consumption.

Using a willing unquestioning media, local celebrities, and scare tactics, marketing campaigns assert that dairy consumption will help reverse the pending osteoporosis "epidemic". In a highly successful move, New Zealand's dairy industry giant Fonterra has aligned itself with General Electric (the manufacturer of Lunar DXA machines) and conducted more than 4 million free bone density scans in Asia and the Middle East since 2005 - an exercise they claim has identified 40 per cent of people tested across Asia to be at a moderate-to-high risk of developing osteoporosis [35]. Such has been the success of Fonterra's Asian campaigns, by 2010 dairy exports account for a full 26 percent of the total goods exported from New Zealand [36].

Frightened women who have had their bone density tested are easily convinced to buy conveniently packed daily 'doses' of Anlene fortified milk, also available reduced to a supposedly palatable 'nutraceutical' form. But changing a diet that has traditionally proven to be beneficial raises many questions, particularly ethical ones, when there is no evidence that dairy consumption will even prevent fracture.

As Hong Kong has undergone increasing urbanization, hip fractureshave increased to the point of doubling in the last 50 years. The reasons given for this are low calcium, lack of exercise, cigarette smoking, alcoholism, and the increasing use of oral and inhaled steroids [37]. Much of Asian urbanization involves the adoption of Western foods and lifestyle trends. Accordingly, the "Western" diseases of breast and prostate cancer are on the rise in countries like Hong Kong and Singapore. Hong Kong now has three times the rate of breast cancer of

MainlandChina. A study of Japanese women who had immigrated to the United States found that when Western-style diet and lifestyle were adopted, the incidence of estrogen-dependent cancers like breast cancer increased [38].

A new study of hip fracture rates in from Beijing from 1990 to 2006 reports a massive 82 percent increase in hip fracture incidence for women aged 70-80 years and an astonishing 442 percent increase for women over the age of 85 years, with similar increases in older men. A doubling in population over 65 years and an increasingly sedentary lifestyle are cited as contributing factors [39].

In 2001 my friend Diane, spent three months as a voluntary primary nurse in the villages of southeast Cambodia, near the border with Vietnam. The villagers would queue to see her every day. She reports having seen no evidence of osteoporosis in the elderly population. She also confirms a total lack of dairy product in the diet of these rural people. "Even the buffalo are not milked. The diet is quite simply rice, vegetables and meat. Other than the availability of yogurt in some supermarkets in Phnom Penh, dairy food is not in evidence."

There's Milk, and There's Milk

Milk may not be the healthy food we think it is. A few facts:

> * Dairy products, with the exception of skim milk products, are loaded with saturated fat. Fat is directly related to heart disease and cancer.
> * Dairy products are very high in protein, which is linked to calcium loss.
> * Prostate cancer and Parkinson's disease in men may be linked to excessive milk consumption [40] [41].
>
> * Many people are allergic to milk, and others are unable to digest the milk sugar lactose and are lactose intolerant [42,43].

Because of the artificial, high-pressure environment they are forced to live in, and without their calves, which are slaughtered at birth, milking cows have a high incidence of mastitis and other infections. For this reason, cows are routinely fed antibiotics. These are then passed directly on to the milk drinkers. A 1990 FDA survey found antibiotics and other drugs in 51 percent of milk samples taken in 14 cities [44]. In her book *Your Life In Your Hands*, Professor Jane Plant observes that "even in the European Union, milk for human consumption can be sold legally even when it contains up to 400,000 somatic pus cells/ml. So one teaspoon of milk can contain 2 million pus cells [45]."

For Americans there is an even greater concern. The United States is the only developed nation to permit humans to consume milk from cows injected with the genetically engineered bovine growth hormone (rBGH). Given to increase milk production, the hormone was banned from use in Canada, Australia, New Zealand, Japan and all European Union countries by 2000 or earlier.

The milk of cows injected with rBGH has higher levels of insulin-like growth factor 1 (IGF-1) than normal milk. Elevated levels of IGF1 in human blood have been linked to increased rates of breast, colon, and prostate cancer [46][47].

The FDA does not require special labels for products produced from cows given rBGH, but consumer demand has led many food chains to label untreated milk, This practice is aggressively contested by rBGH manufacturer Monsanto who claim there is no difference between treated and untreated milk.

In September 2010, a US court of appeal found a "compositional difference" between milk from rBGH-treated cows and untreated milk based on studies showing that rBGH milk has increased levels of the hormone IGF-1; lower nutritional quality when produced at certain points in the cow's lactation cycle; and more pus in the milk [48]. As aresult of continued consumer pressure, approximately 60 percent of milk in the U.S. is rBGH-free in 2010. Many of the contaminants and risks can be avoided by drinking organic milk.

Calcium or not?

Calcium is an essential nutrient. While it is uncertain how much calcium is actually needed, it is certain that diet affects calcium balance. Calcium supplements are not the best way to control osteoporosis for most people. A diet that is modest in protein, high in vegetables, and complemented by exercise is much more effective. Green, leafy vegetables and beans are good sources of calcium that are also moderate in protein and very low in fat. Dark green vegetables, such as broccoli and collard, mustard, and turnip greens are much better sources of calcium than milk. A single cup of broccoli contains almost one-fourth of the U.S. recommended daily amount of calcium. Remember, though, that real requirements may vary depending on the amount of protein and salt that is eaten, and on vitamin D levels. Some twenty minutes of sunlight on the skin every day should produce all the vitamin D the body needs. People who get little or no sun exposure, or who are older, may need a vitamin D supplement. (For more on calcium-rich foods, and food sources of other essential bone nutrients, see Chapter 10.)

Calcium is not a stand-alone issue in maintaining bone health. It is not a magic bullet to target and eliminate the disease known as osteoporosis. Bone needs are complex from a nutritional standpoint.

Calcium is but one of the needs, and its levels may be very dependent on the rest of the composition of the diet. Focusing just on calcium and assuming that dairy is good for you because it contains calcium is just too simple a solution. It is unfortunately one of the most well promoted myths in the osteoporosis story.

***

SECTION III: CREATING BONE HEALTH

***

Chapter 8
Understanding Health

A holistic approach

Frail health, more than any other single factor, leads to bone fractures, which is why maintaining good health is fundamental to creating strong bones and preventing fractures later in life. Staying well means more than taking a prescription drug or mineral supplement. The influences on a woman's health are many, and include nutrition and dietary choices, environmental factors, exercise habits, psychological state and genetic makeup. Some influences we have no control over — we each are born with a unique genetic predisposition to certain diseases or health risks. But in the majority of other areas of our lives, we can control our health.

Creating overall health starts from the day we are born, and lasts until the day we die. The air we breathe, the water we drink, the food we eat, the amount of exercise we undertake, the amount of sleep we get — all of these things influence our health. When the body is young, it has a tremendous ability to heal and repair; people can get away with ingesting junk food, functioning on little rest, ignoring exercise, drinking too much, and smoking. Such habits don't appear to affect the body too badly. But they do.

Once a woman reaches perimenopause, her body quickly lets her know what her limits are, and if she is wise, she will take heed of the signals it gives her. Menopause gives women an opportunity to make significant lifestyle changes in order to stay healthy through the transition and healthy after menopause —

mentally, emotionally, and physically. Every aspect of our health is connected, and if one aspect of ourselves is out of balance, then it affects every part of us.

Linda was diagnosed with osteopenia at age 45. She was initially shocked, then worried, especially when her doctor explained that she stood to lose more bone density as she went through menopause. Linda had practiced yoga and meditation all her life, eaten a largely organic, mineral-rich diet, and worked as a physiotherapist, so she was well informed about the importance of staying flexible and fit. After seeking several opinions and determining that she had no secondary health problems that were contributing to her condition, Linda concluded that she had two choices: Take hormone replacement therapy to further limit bone loss for the duration of the menopause transition, or focus on staying well and fit. She chose the latter and continued her holistic approach to managing her bone health and her life. She educated herself fully about her options, and what her diagnosis could mean, and understood that there are no predictions, no definitive answers, and no magic-bullet solutions. She decided to take responsibility for her future by doing everything she could to maintain good health. It is now five years since her diagnosis and Linda continues to exercise, eat organic foods, and meditatesregularly. She feels very well and has not had a fracture. She no longer feels concerned about her bone density.

The following strategies for a long and healthy life are fundamental to maintaining good bone health and good overall health.

Receiving Adequate Nutrition

Nutrition plays a pivotal role in determining bone health and hip fracture risk. Many elderly people fail to receive adequate intakes of most nutrients, and malnutrition is much worse in those who suffer hip fractures. Several studies have noted that elderly patients, when they are admitted to hospitals with hip fractures, usually have poor nutritional health. A study of 2,500 white women showed that those who had poor nutrition had a significantly higher rate of hip fracture [1].

Japanese women have the highest life expectancy in the world, as well as a low incidence of breast cancer, heart disease, and hip fractures — a fact many researchers attribute to their low-fat, high-fiber diet rich in minerals, vitamins, anti-oxidants and phytoestrogens (plant substances with estrogen-like effects). Japanese women gain these benefits by consuming an abundance of fresh fruits and vegetables, legumes, whole grains, and seafood.

Maintaining Normal Weight

Some women develop a lifelong tendency to diet, trying to attain a standard of beauty defined by a thin-is-better culture. Many well-controlled studies have shown that when a woman loses weight, regardless of age, she loses bone density [2]. Women who diet and exercise to the point of interrupting their menstrual cycles are also known to lose bone density and even fracture [3].

Exercise

The importance of exercise cannot be overstated. Weight-bearing exercise increases bone strength and helps the entire body stay fit. A little exercise goes a long way. Walking for 30 minutes three or four times per week can substantially increase bone strength. Exercise will be discussed in greater detail in the following chapter on creating strong bones.

Avoiding Smoking and Alcohol

Smoking damages the bones as well as the heart and lungs. A study of 300 healthy, young women aged 20 to 29 found that smokers had significantly lower spine BMD and a tendency for lower BMD at other sites [4]. According to a 2001 report, postmenopausal women who smoke cigarettes are significantly more likely to sustain a hip fracture than those who don't smoke [5]. Smokers also may absorb less calcium from their diets [6].

Alcohol has been linked to reduced bone mass because it disrupts the absorption of calcium. The effect is believed to be significant at levels of more than two drinks per day of spirits, beer, or wine. Chronic alcoholism, particularly in men, significantly increases osteoporosis and fractures of the rib, hip, and spine [7].

However, a French study involving 7,500 women over the age of 75 found that drinking one to three glasses of wine each day may have a positive effect on bone mass. The authors caution that nutritional and physical exercise factors were likely to be involved in the outcome of the study, so it couldn't be entirely attributed to the alcohol [8].

Job Satisfaction and Personal Happiness

Doing what you love to do in life will bring you happiness, motivation, and probably success. It will also make you energetic and highly resistant to aging and disease. Discovering what you most enjoy, and doing it, is one of the most powerful techniques for a long and healthy life. Medicine acknowledges that our mind and body operate inseparably, and for this reason it makes sense to look for happiness in whatever we pursue.

Happiness has even been shown to cure life-threatening disease. Norman Cousins, a leader in America's intellectual community in 1964, developed the severe condition of ankylosing spondylitis, a painful, progressive, rheumatic disease affecting the spine and other joints, tendons, and ligaments. He had a tremendous will to live and set himself the task of mobilizing all the natural resources of his body and mind to combat the disease. He rejected conventional treatment and instead forged ahead with a self-prescribed regimen built on high doses of both vitamin C and laughter. He enjoyed a steady diet of "Candid Camera" television episodes and Marx Brothers' films. He found that 10 minutes of genuine belly laughter had an anesthetic effect that would give him least two hours of pain-free sleep. Cousins recovered and more than 10 years later wrote about his recovery in a landmark article in The New England Journal of Medicine and a book, *Anatomy of an Illness* [9]. His breakthrough generated an unprecedented interest in mind-body medicine.

Managing Stress

The tensions and pressures of life generate stress. Levels of the stress hormone cortisol produced by the adrenal glands rise when we are under stress, then fall when the stress disappears. But chronic stress, a common phenomenon in Western life, can override our body's natural ability to bounce back. Sustained stress keeps cortisol levels high, which in turn suppresses our immune response.

If we continue to live in stressful circumstances, we are more likely to develop numerous disorders including infections, obesity, poor wound healing, decreased learning and memory skills, hypertension, stroke, heart attacks, and even osteoporosis (low BMD).

High levels of cortisol can result in the extraction of calcium from our bones, and its circulation back into the blood stream. This means that an excess of cortisol will cause bone loss and ultimately could cause fragile bones. Cortisol can directly suppress production of the hormones DHEA and progesterone and can also suppress thyroid activity. These hormones are all involved in regulating bone turnover. Magnesium deficiency could also be a result of stress; magnesium is essential for normal bone metabolism. Adrenaline, which is also released by the adrenal glands when we are stressed, draws magnesium out of the cells and allows it to be flushed out in the urine [10].

Good health is dependent on managing stress. Research indicates that regular daily exercise, a positive workplace, good friendships, and a spiritual dimension to life are helpful. The practice of meditation is also known to reduce stress levels, improve health and well being. Studies have shown that individuals who have been practicing the technique of Transcendental Meditation (TM) for 20 minutes twice daily for five or more years use hospital services 50 percent less and have an average biological age 12 years younger than their chronological age [11].

Avoiding Exposure to Chemical Pollution

There is preliminary evidence from two studies — one from Sweden and one from Australia — that exposure to the banned pesticide DDT may affect bone mineral density and possibly increase the risk for fragility fractures. The studies were prompted by research two decades ago that showed DDT affected the fertility of birds and made their eggshells lighter [12]. In the human body, DDT metabolizes into DDE, which is known to affect human hormones. A study of 90 women aged 45 to 65 in northern New South Wales found that those with traces of pesticide in their blood had lower bone density than those with none [13]. A group of 115 men from the general Swedish population, ranging in age from 40 to 75 years old, were similarly tested, and a weak association was found between DDE levels and low bone density [14].

Because DDT was used widely as a pesticide from the 1950s to the 1970s, these groups of women and men could have been exposed to it at the time when spraying was at its height, and when peak bone mass was being achieved. DDT has a long half-life in the body — about 72 years — so traces are still detectable, even though spraying is no longer permitted in these countries.

The findings of the two initial studies must be confirmed by larger studies. The preliminary research, however, serves as another salutary reminder that hormone-mimicking environmental chemicals (organochlorines) may be harming our health. Organochlorines are also created by motor vehicle emissions, industrial processes and wastes, pesticides and herbicides. Researchers are finding these chemicals in waterways, soils, and, increasingly, food. Consequently, our bodies are under constant assault from the resulting free radicals (unstable oxygen molecules), which damage cells and are believed to be the root cause of many diseases and chronic illnesses. Since 1980, the incidence of cancer alone has increased by 50 percent in industrialized countries, and from one person in 10 in 1950 to one person in three in 2000. Researchers link the increased incidence of cancer to exposure to carcinogens in the air, water, workplace, or in consumer products [15].

Some of this damage can be averted through the powerful neutralizing effects of naturally occurring dietary antioxidants or free-radical scavengers in fresh fruits and vegetables, and a supplementation with vitamin C and vitamin E. The consumption of organic foods and avoidance of exposure to chemicals is fundamental to reducing the risk of disease from a toxic environment.

Summary

Creating bone health means creating overall health, not just taking a drug or a nutritional supplement. The following chapters outline what you can do to optimize your health, build strong bones, and avoid fracture. They offer concrete steps you can take if you are concerned about osteoporosis and bone health.

***

Chapter 9
Positive Reactions

What to do if you have been given a diagnosis of low bone density.

The rush to measure bone density in apparently healthy women has placed many of them in a difficult situation. What do they do when their test results show that they have low bone density? Many physicians accept unquestioningly that a low bone density reading is a precursor to a disabling fracture and reach for their prescription pads, believing this is the best thing they can do for their patients. Chances are, however, that it is not.

For women who have been given a diagnosis of low bone density, the following three steps can help relieve some of the fear and anxiety.

First, find out what the test results mean. What are your actual risks for having a fracture, especially a hip fracture? Perspective helps. Bone density test results are conveyed in terms of a T-score, a number that rates bone mineral density as compared to a benchmark figure based on healthy, young women in their 20s and 30s — leaving the majority of women with test results that appear abnormal. Instead of looking at your T-score, ask what your Z-score is, a bone mineral density rating based on women your own age. It will give you a more realistic analysis of your bone health. You can also use this information with the questions and tables below to gain an accurate assessment of your risk for hip fracture.

Second, make sure some other medical condition is not causing your low bone density. Some typical tests for this are described below and in depth in Chapter 4.

Third, take steps to minimize the risk of falling. These steps will do more to prevent hip fractures than any other measure.

Fourth, improve your bone health. You can slow bone loss and increase bone strength without medication, as discussed in Chapter 10.

Whether you are at low risk or high risk, these steps will help your bones and your overall health. Recognize that many well women are diagnosed with osteoporosis or osteopenia based solely on the redefinition of the disease as a measure of low bone density. Bone density, however, is only one aspect of bone strength. Other factors are much more important in determining fracture risk.

Understanding Your Risk of Fracture

Age is an important factor in understanding your risk of fracture. A 50-year-old woman is very unlikely to have a fracture related to osteoporosis, whereas a 90-year-old woman has a 30 percent chance of breaking her hip. Age is an important factor in deciding what your next step will be.

Another important determinant is whether you have had a fracture since your 50th birthday. A personal history of low-trauma fracture is one of the most important risk factors, because it demonstrates that your bones are possibly already fragile, not just that they have the potential to be. "Low trauma" means fracturing a bone with minimal impact. The presence of a spinal fracture is also an important predictor of future fracture.

In assessing risk, family history is a strong determining factor, especially immediate family. If your mother has fractured her hip, that will increase your likelihood of fracture. Other factors also play an important role, such as:

1) Sedentary Lifestyle — *A sedentary lifestyle can cause bone loss. Regular exercise sustains bone remodeling and helps prevent falls in the elderly.*

2) Smoking — *Smokers are more at-risk than nonsmokers because of the tendency to have lower bone density, lower body weight, and lower estrogen levels.*

3) Low Body Weight — *This is a strong predictor of fracture risk. Research indicates that a weight of 132 pounds or more offers protection. Weight loss is associated with significant BMD loss in postmenopausal women, and many experts advise against constant dieting. Conversely, small bones automatically register lower on bone density tests even if they are not thinner, which can make small bones look more at risk than they are.*

4) Loss of Height — *Find out if there has been height loss and how much. Loss of height can be related to compression of discs, but a loss of height of more than 3 centimeters (about 1.2 inches) usually indicates vertebral deformity.*

5) Early or Surgical Menopause — This can cause increased bone loss in some women.

6) Cessation of Periods — If your period has stopped for 12 months or more (other than because of pregnancy), you may be at greater risk. Eating disorders, over-exercising, and emotional trauma may interfere with normal menstruation. This can influence bone remodeling and cause reduced bone density

7) Prescription Medications — Certain drugs like corticosteroids are associated with bone loss and increased rate of fracture. (See full list of drugs at the end of Chapter 4.)

Certain diseases that cause frequent diarrhea are associated with osteoporosis, such as celiac disease or Crohn's disease.

Understanding the factors that can increase your risk of fracture will help you to put your test results in perspective. Another way of doing this is to try to quantify your risk, as the next section explains.

Assessing Your Risk of Hip Fracture

Hip fractures are the most debilitating fractures — and should therefore be the target of preventative strategies. Assessing your actual risk of hip fracture can determine whether you need to be concerned and consider aggressive treatment, or whether your risks are minimal and you can rest at ease.

A 1995 study published in the New England Journal of Medicine followed more than 9,000 women to determine which risk factors are significant in determining a risk for hip fracture [1]. The results showed that bone density was only one of several factors that have to be taken into account, and that low bone density only became a cause for concern in the presence of a least five other risk factors. The factors that significantly contributed to hip fracture risk are outlined below. To approximate your actual risk of hip fracture, put a check by the risk factors you have and total the number of checks.

1. Age greater than 80.	☐
2. History of hip fracture in your mother.	☐
3. Any fracture (except hip fracture) since age 50.	☐
4. Fair, poor, or very poor health (as opposed to good or excellent health).	☐
5. Previous history of hyperthyroidism.	☐
6. Taking seizure medication.	☐
7. Taking long-acting tranquilizers (benzodiazepenes).	☐
8. Current weight less than it was at age 25.	☐
9. Height at age 25 greater than 5 feet 6 inches tall.	☐
10. Caffeine intake more than the equivalent of two cups of coffee per day.	☐
11. On feet 4 hours a day or less.	☐
12. Do not walk for exercise.	☐
13. Cannot rise from a chair without using your arms.	☐
14. Poor depth perception – the ability to see objects in perspective.	☐
15. Difficulty seeing contrasts.	☐
16. Resting pulse rate is greater than 80 beats per minute.	☐
TOTAL ____	

After you have determined your number of risk factors, use this information together with your bone density testing results (your Z-scores, if you have them) to get an approximation of your risk. If you are not sure where your testing results fall, ask your health-care provider whether your results fall in the lowest, middle, or upper third *for women your age*. The chart below determines the percent of women like you who will have a hip fracture within the next 10 years, when they become 72. *

HIGHEST THIRD BONE DENSITY (Z-score >= 0.43)
If your bone density is in the highest third for women your age, and your number of risk factors is:
0 - 2: Your risk is 1.1 percent
3 - 4: Your risk is 1.9 percent
5 or greater: Your risk is 9.4 percent
MIDDLE THIRD (AVERAGE) BONE DENSITY (Z-score -0.42 to +0.42)
If your bone density is in the middle third for women your age, and your number of risk factors is:
0 - 2: Your risk is 1.1 percent
3 - 4: Your risk is 5.6 percent
5 or greater: Your risk is 14.7 percent
LOWEST THIRD BONE DENSITY (Z-score <= -0.43)
If your bone density is in the lowest third for women your age, and your number of risk factors is:
0 - 2: Your risk is 2.6 percent
3 - 4: Your risk is 4.0 percent
5 or greater: Your risk is 27.3 percent

Estimated percent of women who will have a hip fracture within the next 10 years, starting at age 72*

*The study participants had an average age of 72. The following chart can be used as an approximation only, because the study group may have different characteristics from you. In addition, the original data was reported as annual risk per 1,000 women-years, and has been transformed to percent risk per 10 years to make the approximation of risk more easily understood.

Suppose you have a Z-score of -0.2 (middle third) and you have two risk factors — your height is greater than 5 feet 6 inches and your resting pulse rate is 82 beats per minute. From the chart, you can see that your risk of fracture is 1.1 percent. If you were to take drugs to increase your bone density to the highest third, your risk for fracture would not change. To greatly reduce the risk of fracture, people need to reduce the number of risk factors. People who have five or more risk factors need to consider making lifestyle changes to improve their health. Many of the risk factors, such as "not walking for exercise," can be changed without medications. Note also that bone density doesn't play a major role until a person has *five or more* risk factors.

In assessing your osteoporosis risk, other factors may also need to be taken into account. For example, if you smoke or take medications like corticosteroids, your risk is increased. If you have had an early menopause or surgical menopause, your risk may also be increased.

Checking for Other Causes

If your bone density is very low (or even if your bone density is normal), and you want to eliminate other risk factors, then ask your doctor for the following tests:

* If you have lost height and if your DXA scan shows low BMD in the spine, then a lateral spine X-ray will determine whether there has been any compression fracturing.

* Blood (serum) vitamin D and calcium levels.

* A thyroid test — especially if there is a family history of hypothyroidism or hyperthyroidism.

* A 24-hour calcium/urine test will measure how much calcium is being lost in the urine. If there are high levels of calcium in the urine, then you need to see a specialist.

* DXA scan in more than one bone site. It is possible that there can be some inaccuracies with DXA scanning, particularly if you have already had a

spinal fracture that has caused some compression in your vertebrae. This can make your bones seem denser than they are. Sometimes, fractures of the vertebrae go unnoticed, as they can be painless. Measuring the hip as well can give a more accurate reading.

* A bone marker urine test can gauge the approximate rate of bone breakdown or bone resorption by measuring the breakdown products of collagen. It is normally quite high postmenopause, but repeat testing every three to six months will indicate whether bone loss is occurring. The tests to request are Dpd, or deoxypyridinoline, and NTx, or N-telopeptide, which measure bone breakdown or resorption, and bone alkaline phosphatase (ALP), which measures bone formation.

* Celiac disease. There are three antibody blood tests that, if all are positive, indicate a high probability of celiac disease. The tests are: endomysial, reticulin (Inga), and gliadin (Gig and Inga) antibodies.

* For men, serum testosterone levels could also be measured.

* Have blood levels of magnesium, zinc, manganese, boron, and other trace minerals tested.

Preventing Falls

As we age, muscle mass naturally decreases, skin becomes thinner, and fat shifts to the center of the body — physical changes that decrease the body's ability to pad itself in the event of a fall and prevent fractures. Therefore, regardless of bone density, people must take extra care to avoid falls as they age. Studies show that fall-prevention strategies significantly reduce the incidence of hip fractures. The following steps can help reduce the risk of falling:

1. Maintain a Safe Home

The home can be a hazardous place. Many falls occur as a result of obstacles such as loose floor rugs and mats, electrical cords, and poorly placed furniture. Suggestions:

* Have your home assessed for risk by an occupational therapist.
* Install handrails around steps and stairs, in the bathroom by the shower and toilet, and outside at any entrance to your

house.
* Cover steps and stairs with nonslip material.
* Remove all loose rugs, and secure carpets with nonskid tape.
* Do not polish or wax floors.
* Remove extension cords.
* Clear clutter so that you can move easily from room to room.
* Arrange furniture such as coffee tables so you can move around easily.
* Check that lighting is adequate and effective.
* Install an emergency response system.
* Have telephone extensions in each main area.
* Use a cordless telephone where possible.

The bathroom is the most dangerous room in the house. Suggestions:
* Remove loose bathmats.
* Use nonskid mats, abrasive strips, and grab bars in showers and tubs.
* Ensure lighting is adequate.
* Make sure toilet seats are not wobbly and are high enough.

The kitchen is the second-most dangerous room. Suggestions:

* Ensure lighting is more than adequate.
* Rearrange cupboards so that you don't have to reach or bend far for commonly used items.
* Put appliance cords well out of the way.
* Use a sturdy step stool with handrails.
* Clean up spills from floors immediately.

Bedroom, living room, and hallway floors are dangerous areas with many minor dangers that can become major hazards. Suggestions:
* Remove clutter.
* Remove loose mats and rugs.
* Have bright lights in stairways and hallways.
* Install strong handrails running the length of halls and stairs.
* Raise beds and chairs to a height that is easy to get into and out of.
* Remove caster wheels from furniture.
* Have a bedside lamp that is easy to reach and turn on.
* Install a night light.
* Have telephone within easy reach of bed.
* Watch out for pets – they can get underfoot and cause a fall.

2. Understand the Side Effects of Any Medication You Take

Certain medications such as sedatives, antidepressants, and antipsychotic drugs can cause dizziness, drowsiness, and blurred vision, which can lead to falling. Medications can also reduce alertness, affect balance and gait, and cause a sudden drop in blood pressure when standing or rising from a chair. People taking multiple medications are at greater risk of falling.

Suggestions:
* Discuss the side effects and interactions of your medications with your physician or pharmacist.
* Request the lowest effective dose.
* If you see more than one physician, make sure that each one knows all the medication you are taking.
* Take all your medications with you when you visit the doctor.

* Get rid of all out-of-date medications.
* Make sure all medications are clearly labeled and stored in a well-lit area.
* Use walking aids, if using medications that affect balance.
* Get up slowly when lying down or sitting

up if you have heart problems or high blood pressure.

* Talk to your doctor about managing poor bladder control to avoid rushing to the restroom.
* Limit alcohol intake. Drinking can make you unsteady and it can interact with medications.

3. Maintain Your Eyesight Poor vision is associated with an increased risk for falling. Suggestions:

* Have annual checkups with your eye doctor to monitor for conditions such as glaucoma and cataracts.
* Keep eyeglasses clean.
* Add contrasting color strips to handrails and steps in the home.

4. Wear Sturdy Footwear and Reduce Environmental Hazards

* Wear low-heeled, supportive shoes with rubber soles.
* Avoid loose slippers, shoes with leather soles, or high heels.
* Never walk in your stocking feet.
* Avoid uneven walking surfaces, broken or cracked sidewalks, and construction areas.
* Park your car where it is clear of snow

and ice.
* Avoid wet surfaces.
* Install sensor lights outdoors that will turn on whenever there is motion.

5. Wear Hip Protectors

Thinner and frail women have less fat and soft tissue to protect them when they fall. Elderly people who are at high risk for fracture can wear a padded undergarment to absorb the energy of a high-impact fall and reduce the risk of hip fracture. There is evidence that the pads can reduce hip fracture rates by half.

Taking Positive Action to Create Bone Health

Many of the risk factors for fractures involve lifestyle choices that you can control and modify. The next chapter explains how to decrease your risks, and take positive action to increase bone density and create better health.

***

Chapter 10
Creating Strong Bones

What every woman should know.

My parents lead active lives and keep good health. My father is in his mid-90s and my mother her late 80s. They have been married for 65 years. They have a large property, grow vegetables, and enjoy a beautiful flower garden. They are still actively involved in church and community projects and take great interest in each member of our large extended family. My mother sustained several painful vertebral fractures in her mid-80s followed by a bad fall on the side-walk which fractured her shoulder, resulting in a shoulder replacement procedure, Although she has lost considerable height she recovered well from these setbacks and was able to resume her normal active life. Then very recently she fractured a hip after tripping over a wheel stop in a car park. She has made a remarkable recovery following a partial hip replacement. She is able to walk well, is pain free, and was driving again after six weeks. My mother continues to cook healthy meals and run the household. She is highly organized and has good physical stamina. She also has been the "eyes" for two people since my father lost his sight 24 years ago.

My father served in the New Zealand army medical corps in Italy and Egypt during World War II and has been physically fit all his life. He exercises daily – specifically weight bearing and back strengthening exercises. He has never fractured. My parents exemplify the way in which simple lifestyle choices can help people live longer, healthier, and happier lives. Exercising on a regular basis and eating healthy foods are two of the best ways to maintain good health and create excellent bone health.

Exercise

Study after study shows that moderate exercise helps to prevent a host of chronic illnesses, from diabetes to heart disease to osteoporosis. Exercise benefits the skeleton, and is the single most effective strategy to prevent fragility fracture. No other agent, hormonal or mineral, can actually cause the skeleton to become heavier or sturdier in response to the demands made of it. Bone formation is stimulated by the mechanical forces that exercise generates, particularly higher-impact activities like jogging, running, and jumping that generate more effect on bones than lower-impact exercise like swimming or walking.

The force of muscles pulling against bones promotes new bone growth, and the more you use your muscles, the more this stimulates bone remodeling and bone formation. This effect has been repeatedly observed in athletes. A recent study of volleyball players demonstrated that top male volleyball players show remarkably high bone density in the hip and spine regions, and high bone density in their arms and legs. Interestingly, the arm used to spike the volleyball was up to 9 percent more dense than the less-involved arm, believed to be a result of the body's adaptation to the greater demands made on that arm [1].

A review of all the randomized controlled studies done on exercise and bone mass in pre and postmenopausal women concluded that exercise prevented or reversed about onepercent of bone loss per year at the spine and the hip [2]. There is also evidence that women with the lowest BMD tend to show the greatest response to exercise — a great incentive for anyone with a BMD diagnosis of osteoporosis [3].

When it comes to exercise, age is no barrier. People more than 80 years old can reduce their risk of osteoporosis while also improving muscle tone and balance [4]. Exercise programs offered by trained health professionals that target strength and balance, or strength and endurance, have been found to reduce the frequency of falls in high-risk, older people. These specific exercise programs incorporate walking, the gentle and gradual use of weights, and exercises to increase balance. A New Zealand home exercise program delivered by trained nurses to 450 women and men aged 79 to 94 resulted in a 30 percent reduction in the incidence of falls [5].

Coincidentally, my father participated in this program. He followed the exercise routines daily for several months and significantly increased the amount of weight he could lift and the duration of use. Soon after the program ended, he underwent a major surgical procedure. His excellent recovery could in part be attributed to the level of strength and fitness achieved at the time.

Physical activity is one of the most important factors in acquiring peak bone mass during youth. Many researchers believe that as children and young adults log increasing numbers of hours watching television and sitting in front of computers, their bone mass may be suffering for it. High impact exercise has been found to have the most beneficial effect on bone mass in girls before puberty, rather than after [6].

Regular exercise has numerous other benefits. It increases well being and fitness. It also helps protect against conditions like heart disease, cancer, depression, and Alzheimer's disease [7]. In addition, weight training can give a sense of competency when daily tasks such as lifting, carrying groceries, or pushing the lawn mower become much easier. Although weight training is not aerobic, it helps increase metabolism, which can help shed excess weight.

Sedentary Lives

Lack of exercise and immobility will reduce bone density, general strength, and fitness. Bedridden patients lose muscle and bone, and have increased levels of urinary calcium, indicating that calcium is being lost from the bone.

A survey of adult New Zealanders revealed that they spend an average of 40 minutes a day on grooming, an hour and a half socializing, an hour and a half eating, two hours watching TV and eight minutes exercising [8]. Most likely this is similar throughout the developed nations. Life in the 21stcentury works against us being physically active. In fact, it continues to get easier to avoid exercising. Daily activity is geared toward working our bodies less and less, as technology replaces physical effort. Many of us sit for hours in front of computer screens and now send mostof our mail electronically — denyingus even the walk to the mailbox. We drive from destination to destination — no matter how short the drive; and when we arrive, escalators and elevators lift us from floor to floor.

The National Aeronautics and Space Administration physicians discovered astronauts lost bone in space at the rate of 1.5 percent per month. Dr. Norman Thagard spent 115 days in space on the Russian space station Mir. He lost 11.7 percent of his bone density and 17.5 pounds of overall muscle and weight during his sojourn. Most of this loss came from the hip and lower spine. Dr. Frank M. Sulzman, director of life science research at NASA, says a trip to Mars, which is estimated to take between one and two years each way, may leave an astronaut permanently crippled upon return to Earth [9].

No group is at higher risk for depression, disease, and early death than people who are completely sedentary. Studies from the Russian space program also showed that young cosmonauts subjected to the forced inactivity of space flight fell prey to depression. When they were put on a schedule of regular exercise, the depression was avoided [10].

Exercise and the Older Person

Physiologists used to believe that exercise primarily benefited us at young ages when muscles are in their prime developmental stage. However, research with the elderly has conclusively demonstrated that a person can take up exercise at any age — even centenarians will receive the same increase in strength, stamina, and muscle mass. Weight training, in particular, has special benefits for the frail elderly. In a 1992 study of frail, very old volunteers who were prone to falling easily, Maria Fiatarone and colleagues at the Hebrew Rehabilitation Center for Aged observed that, after adopting a regular resistance training program, men and women tripled their thigh muscle mass and dramatically lowered their risk of falls [11].

An Oregon State University study found that older women who participated in a long-term fitness regimen that included jumping and "resistance" exercises using weighted vests showed a reduction in significant bone loss in the hip. Some participants even showed an increase in bone density. The exercise program developed by Christine Snow had already been shown to be effective in helping the elderly reduce their risk of falls by improving their strength and balance [12].

And researchers from Tufts University showed that elderly nursing home residents, ranging in age from 86 to 96, dramatically increased their strength and improved their balance after just eight weeks of supervised weight training. Now studies have proved that working out with free weights or machines can help restore lost bone density, as well as reduce knee pain from arthritis and keep the body sensitive to the insulin it produces to keep sugar levels in balance [13].

A ten-year follow-up study has found that back extensor-strengthening (BES) exercises reduce the risk of vertebral compression fractures in postmenopausal women. The participants wore a weighted backpack, lay on their stomachs and lifted the backpack ten times 5 days a week for 2 years. As their back strength increased they weight was increased to a maximum of 50 pounds. The study also found that the benefits of weight-bearing exercise could continue even if the exercising stops [14]. And a review of the literature in 2004 concluded that exercise was associated with a reduced risk of hip fracture [15].

There are four main types of exercise :

1. Aerobic
Aerobic exercise increases cardiovascular function and strength. Walking is great aerobic exercise that stimulates the leg and hip bones by the impact of your feet hitting the ground. There is, however, little or no evidence that aerobic exercise alone will increase bone density.

2. Flexibility
Stretching exercises promote flexibility, which helps to prevent falls. Having strong and flexible joints also means that you are less likely to suffer joint injuries. Yoga is excellent in this regard. It is weight-bearing exercise, and in the various yoga postures, the muscles pull on the bone stimulating further remodeling.

3. Balance Training
As we age our sense of balance becomes less, and as a consequence, we are more at risk of falling. Balance training occurs in Tai Chi or other programs like Pilates that are specially designed to improve balance and core strength.

Visit a local park in the early morning in China and you will see older men and women practicing Tai Chi, a series of postures and exercises characterized by slow, relaxing, and graceful movements. Tai Chi enhances balance and body awareness. Legend has it that in the 12th century, a group of Chinese monks decided to try a new form of meditation — one that would imitate the rhythms of the world and the life all around them. Tai Chi was the result.

The main principle of Tai Chi is that it uses subtle movements that cause energy to flow in the body. Tai Chi, according to traditional Chinese medicine, is an excellent way of accumulating energy (chi), storing it, and then circulating it through the body. This balances the body and prevents and heals disease. Studies show that Tai Chi can improve strength, flexibility, and endurance in patients suffering from osteoarthritis. It is an excellent weight-bearing exercise, which can decrease joint swelling and tenderness, improve balance, and reduce the incidence of falls in men and women over 70 years old [16].

It is one of the only exercises that teaches how to bear all the body weight on one leg at a time. This promotes increased bone formation in the weight-bearing pelvic bones and femur. A U.S. study of the effect of regular Tai Chi exercises over a 15-week period included 200 participants age 70 and older. The participants were divided into groups for Tai Chi, balance training, and education. The most notable outcome was a 47.5 percent reduction in the rate of multiple falls for the Tai Chi group. Fear of falling was also reduced. The groups receiving balance training and education did not have significantly lower rates of falling [17].

Commentators at the time noted that the success of Tai Chi is a reminder that relatively "low tech" approaches should not be overlooked in the search for ways to prevent disability and maintain physical performance in late life. And it needn't take a lot of time — a mere 10 minutes of Tai Chi practice a day is reported to be beneficial for most people who choose this exercise as a part of their health regimen. Once you have received qualified instruction, you can practice it successfully at home, or in your local park!

4. Resistance or Strength Training

Many studies confirm that strength training by using weights and high-impact exercises can build bone. As muscles contract when we lift weights, they pull on the bone to which they are attached, which then stimulates the bone to build in that area. For this reason is it important to practice a range of exercises that will stimulate the whole skeleton, particularly those areas at higher risk for fracture.

All four types of exercise are important in maintaining fitness, good health, and preventing osteoporosis. But for exercise to be most effective in preventing or slowing bone loss, it must stress the skeleton. As long as exercise does not involve any sudden or excessive strain on the bones and is compatible with a person's general health, then the more exercise the better, from a skeletal point of view. Many experts recommend that people alternate their exercise routine so that the muscles (and bone) receive a varied workout. The idea is that if you can surprise the bone in the way you load it, you may continue to stimulate more bone mineralization and bone strengthening.

A heavier weight lifted fewer times is better than a lighter load lifted more often. A 1996 exercise study compared two types of strength training regimens, which differed in the number of repetitions and the weights lifted. The strength program that involved heavy amounts of weight with low repetitions significantly increased bone density at the hip and forearm sites, whereas the endurance program that featured lighter amounts of weight and high numbers of repetitions had no effect [18]. Strength training is also important for maintaining muscle strength with aging.

Weight training isolates specific muscle groups in various parts of your body — shoulders, chest, arms, back, legs, and stomach — and works them one at a time. A variety of exercises are available for each muscle group. Most experts recommend that you establish a routine that works all of the different muscle groups at least once during the course of a week. It is also advisable to change your weight-training routine periodically by trying new exercises that will work the muscles in a slightly different way. The following weight-training exercises that cover all the muscle groups are suggested for healthy adults [19]. It is important always to learn safe lifting techniques. Ask an expert to teach you how to do them.

   Biceps curl
* Overhead press

- Wrist curl
* Reverse wrist curl
* Triceps extension
* Forearm pronation/supination
* Bench press
* Leg press
* Half squats
* Hip abduction/adduction
* Hamstring curl
* Hip flexion
* Hip extension

It is important to understand that a woman's body will respond differently to weight training than a man's because of hormonal differences. The hormone testosterone plays a major role in muscular development. Because women have less of this hormone, they tend not to "bulk-up" with weight training.

How To Get Started

The first word of advice on lifting weights is: "Proceed with caution." It's essential to begin with very light weights — weights that are so easy to lift they seem to be flying through the air. Don't try to prove yourself. Strength comes with time and practice; lifting heavy amounts of weight too early in your regimen can lead to injuries that prevent you from exercising at all.

It's best to follow a routine developed by a qualified training expert who can also demonstrate technique and form. Gyms and health clubs usually have on-site trainers. Many fitness consultants can be hired privately. For the budget-conscious, a trip to the library can be helpful; there is no shortage of fitness books that feature explanations and photos of many exercises. There are several good books and web sites that can also help you get started with your weight-training program.

General Rules for Resistance Training

* Consult your health-care provider before beginning any new exercise program.

* A warm-up is essential and will help prevent injury. Walking in place, stepping, or jumping rope for a few minutes will help get your muscles geared up for action.

* Go slowly. Start with light weights and lift them slowly, in a controlled manner. Do not strain.

* Most experts recommend that you exercise larger muscles groups before smaller ones to achieve maximum benefits. To strengthen the legs, for example, work the quadriceps muscles before the calf muscles.

* Use the same amount of weight in your left and right hands. Even if one side of your body seems to be stronger, be consistent in the amount of weights you use.

* Don't over train. Rest one or two days before exercising the same muscle group a second time.

* Follow the workout instructions and guidelines about the number of times to lift each weight (repetitions), and how many sets of each exercise to do.

* Don't forget to breathe! Keep your muscles oxygenated.

* Stretch at the completion of your workout to help avoid stiffness and injury.

Precautions

It is extremely important that anyone who undertakes strength training is properly supervised to ensure good technique, especially if they have low bone mass. Weight training may be dangerous if performed improperly or without supervision. If you already have osteoporosis, or have had a fragility fracture, it is very important that you avoid high-impact weight lifting, jumping, abrupt or explosive movements, twisting movements, and intense abdominal exercises. Individuals with high blood pressure, back problems, or hernias should consult a physician prior to engaging in a weight-training program.

How Often Should You Exercise?

Most studies show that people who exercise for one hour, two to three times a week, can significantly slow or prevent bone loss — a benefit equivalent to that achieved by people who exercise every day. Experts recommend easing yourself into an exercise program and gradually increasing your routine over time. For elderly or sedentary people, exercise should be gradually introduced to minimize fatigue and sore muscles. It is also important to have variety in the program and make sure that all muscle groups are being exercised. A carefully supervised strength-training program can do that.

Adding weights to the body during aerobic exercise is an excellent way to do at least two forms of exercise simultaneously. Ankle and arm weights that can be purchased for little investment can be worn for short periods during light exercise.

Exercise Summarized

Exercise is the single most important strategy to maintain healthy bones. For exercise to be effective, it must be continued throughout life. If we are immobile or inactive, it will lead to bone loss. Sustained weight-bearing exercise will maintain bone formation and help prevent fracture. Older people who walk and exercise regularly have better coordination, muscle strength, and flexibility — important factors in preventing falls. While exercise is the most important strategy for maintaining healthy bone, dietary and nutritional factors also play a significant role.

Dietary and Nutritional Factors

Diet has a significant effect on bone health, which makes sense, considering the process by which bone is constantly being dissolved and rebuilt involves various nutrients and minerals extracted from the blood supply. Yet, achieving the optimum dietary intake of essential nutrients may not be as easy as eating an apparent "balanced diet."

Many high-protein foods — including meat, eggs, and dairy products — contain rich sources of phosphoric and sulfuric acid. The consumption of such foods, known as "acid ash" foods, will cause acid to form in the body and over time will alter the body's pH balance – which measures the degree of acidity or alkalinity in the blood. As the pH level becomes acidic, the body buffers this by leaching calcium from the bone. Even a small drop in the body's pH can cause a dramatic increase in bone loss [20]. It is advisable to test your urine to determine your pH levels.

If you are too acidic, increasing your intake of alkaline-producing foods — leafy greens, sea vegetables, non-starchy vegetables, nuts and seeds — will create a bone-nutrient rich, pH balancing diet that reduces calcium excretion and bone loss. It can also limit the need for supplements, as these foods are a rich source of vitamins, minerals, and protein. Sea vegetables (seaweeds), for example, contain high amounts of calcium, phosphorus, magnesium, boron, iron, iodine, and sodium.

An investigation of the diets of elderly men and women in Framingham Massachusetts, found that people who ate more fruits and vegetables rich in potassium and magnesium had less bone mass loss in the hip and forearm than those elderly people who ate less of these foods [21]. A follow-up study also found that high fruit and vegetable intake appears to be protective in men, and high candy consumption is associated with low bone mass in both men and women [22].

Protein is also important for bone health, and too little can have an adverse effect on bone. People's protein needs vary, depending on body mass and activity level. Adults are recommended to have approximately 40 to 60 grams of protein daily. Meat, fish, eggs, and milk have large quantities of protein. Vegetable protein is found in grains such as rice and wheat, beans, lentils, nuts and seeds. Pumpkin, squash, and sunflower seeds contain high amounts of protein. They are also most nutritious eaten raw. Flaxseeds and sesame seeds are high in protein and also a good source of calcium. Walnuts, almonds and cashews are the highest in protein of the commonly eaten nuts. Lentils have a lot of protein, while soybeans contain more than twice as much protein as other beans. Other high-protein legumes include garbanzos and black beans.

The typeof protein can affect bone strength. The Study of Osteoporotic Fracture (SOF) trial showed that women who consumed more animal protein than vegetable protein had a higher rate of bone loss at the hip. It also showed a greater risk of hip fracture in women who consumed more animal protein than women who ate vegetable protein [23]. Many experts therefore recommend reducing meat and dairy intake, and increasing vegetable protein consumption.

When meat protein consumption is high, then more calcium is required as well. A 1994 report in the American Journal of Clinical Nutrition showed that when animal proteins were eliminated from the diet, calcium losses were cut in half [24]. Another study followed more than 85,000 American women for 12 years. Those who ate the most animal protein (meat, poultry and dairy) had a significantly higher risk of osteoporotic fractures [25].

Phytoestrogens

Phytoestrogens are plant compounds that have a multitude of hormone-like properties that may be beneficial to women. There is some evidence that regular consumption of fruits, vegetables, grains, and legumes rich in these plant hormones can positively influence a woman's health and hormone balance. Phytoestrogen-rich foods may decrease menopause symptoms including hot flashes, help prevent osteoporosis, and reduce the incidence of heart disease [26, 27, 28].

The traditional diets of approximately half the world's population contain moderate to high levels of phytoestrogens. In Asian cultures, women traditionally have a diet that is low fat, high fiber, and rich in a wide variety of fresh fruit and vegetables (phytoestrogens). This stands in contrast to the high-protein, carbohydrate-rich, fat-based diet more typically found in Western countries. A study of Japanese women who had immigrated to the United States found that when Western-style diet and lifestyle was adopted, the incidence of estrogen-dependent cancers, like breast cancer, increased [31].

Phytoestrogens are found in:

Soy — *tofu, temper, miso, soy milk, soy flour and roasted soybeans, and soy extract powders*
Legumes — *chickpeas, lentils, and many beans including mung, haricot, broad, kidney, and lima*
Wholegrain Cereals — *wheat, wheat*

germ, barley, rye, rice, bran, oats Fruit — cherries, apples, pears, peaches, apricots, plums and other stone fruit, and rhubarb
Seeds — linseed or flaxseed, sunflower, anise, sesame Vegetables — green and yellow vegetables, carrots, fennel, onion, garlic
Vegetable Oils — olive oil
Herbs and Roots — ginseng, licorice, hops

Soy is Controversial

These days, traditional methods of soy preparation involving a long process of fermentation have been abandoned in favor of a quicker form of processing. Soy milk, for example, is produced by soaking the beans in an alkaline solution, then heating them to about 115 degrees Celsius. This produces difficult-to-digest proteins and phytates that can block the essential uptake of minerals. It appears that the traditional methods of preparation reduced soy's mineral-robbing "anti-nutrients," and improved its digestibility. The only modern, commercial soy foods that undergo this fermentation are temper (not tofu) and miss (not soy sauce). While traditionally prepared tofu may be on the market, there is often no distinct labeling to mark it as such.

Soy is also being genetically engineered to be resistant to herbicides, and now floods the global market in its altered form. Genetically engineered foods have been controversial because the effect of this altered genetic material on humans is unknown and untested. To avoid consuming genetically engineered soy, it is necessary to eat products labeled "organic," "GE free," or "No Gomes."

Some experts warn against feeding soy milk to infants, as large quantities of even weak plant hormone may be inappropriate for children. The effect of adding large quantities of soy (particularly soy milk) to the adult diet is also unknown. Some people speculate that because soy foods are relatively new to Western men and women, their digestive systems may not have evolved to cope with them.

Other Dietary Considerations
Sodium (salt)
A definite link between salt intake and fracture risk has not yet been established,

though increases in dietary salt have led to an increase in the loss of calcium in the urine. People who reduce their sodium intake to 1 to 2 grams per day cut their calcium requirement by an average of 60 milligrams per day [34]. Most nutrition experts therefore recommend less salt and less highly salted foods.

Caffeine
Most nutritional experts recommend avoiding coffee or restricting consumption to one cup a day. Coffee is acidic and is therefore linked to increased bone loss, but there is no evidence that it is linked to fragility fractures. In one trial, caffeine was linked with lower bone mass, but only in women who consumed relatively little calcium [35]. The authors of this report conclude that two to three cups of coffee per day might speed bone loss in women with calcium intakes of less than 800 milligrams per day.

Vitamin D
Vitamin D is essential for the normal growth and development of the teeth, bones, and cartilage in children. It's also needed to keep adult teeth in good repair. Vitamin D also prevents osteomalacia, or

rickets, a deficiency disease characterized by malformations of bones and teeth in children, and by brittle, easily broken bones in adults. Age-related vitamin D deficiency leads to malabsorption of calcium, accelerated bone loss, muscle weakness and increased risk for hip fracture. (Read more about vitamin D in Chapter 6.)

Magnesium

Magnesium's role in bone health appears to be significant. As much as 50 percent of the body's magnesium is found in the bones. Magnesium influences bone metabolism and is also important for calcium regulation. (Although the optimum ratio of calcium to magnesium is not established, there is evidence that two parts calcium to one part magnesium will allow for better calcium absorption. Milk apparently has four parts calcium to one part magnesium [36].)

Many researchers are now reporting that magnesium deficiency is common, and that it plays a big part in the development of osteoporosis. A typical American diet contains about 250 milligrams of magnesium, while the U.S. recommended daily allowance (RDA) of magnesium is 350 milligrams. Moreover, some researchers believe that the optimal daily intake of this mineral is more than 600 milligrams. Magnesium is found in many foods (see chart below).

If levels of magnesium become depleted, bone growth stops. A magnesium deficiency can also affect the production of the biologically active form of vitamin D, and thereby further promote osteoporosis. A 1995 review on the role of magnesium states: "There is growing evidence that magnesium may be an important factor in the qualitative changes of the bone matrix that determine bone fragility [37]." The authors of the report note that bone mineral with decreased magnesium content results in larger abnormally shaped bone crystals, which may be more brittle than smaller, normal crystals. They add: "Trabecular bone from osteoporotic women has a reduced magnesium content and larger bone crystal formation than controls."

Studies have shown that women with low bone density tend to have a lower intake of magnesium than normal, and also have lower levels of magnesium in their blood and their bones [38]. A trial in Israel showed that postmenopausal women with osteoporosis (low BMD) could stop further bone loss by supplementing with 250 to 750 milligrams per day of magnesium for two years [39]. Eight percent of the women experienced a significant increase in bone density. Untreated controls lost bone density. Another study in Czechoslovakia found that 65 percent of women who supplemented with 1,500 to 3,000 milligrams of magnesium lactate daily for two years were rid of their pain and stopped further development of deformities of the vertebrae [40].

A 1998 Austrian study of magnesium supplementation in young males found indications that magnesium suppressed high bone turnover, which could be beneficial in reducing associated bone loss [41]. An Australian study investigating how a mother's diet during pregnancy affected her children's BMD, found that spinal bone density was significantly higher with the highest maternal intake of phosphorus, magnesium, and potassium. BMD was lower with a high maternal fat intake. According to the researchers, total body BMD was significantly associated with magnesium only [42].

Calcium

The body needs calcium, preferably from food, as opposed to supplements. Current recommendations range from 1,200 to 1,500 milligrams of calcium per day. The best-absorbed calcium sources are green, leafy vegetables, legumes, and seeds. They have several advantages that dairy products lack. Dairy foods contain animal protein, and havecomparatively low levels of magnesium. Vegetables and legumes contain antioxidants, complex carbohydrates, fiber, and iron, and have little fat and no cholesterol.

The body also absorbs calcium more efficiently when it comes from vegetables rather than dairy products. For example, calcium absorption from milk is approximately 32 percent, while calcium absorption from broccoli, Brussels sprouts, mustard greens, turnip greens, and kale ranges from 40 percent to 64 percent [43]. Spinach is an exception. It contains a large amount of calcium, but in a form that is poorly absorbed due to the presence of oxalic acid. Beans (e.g., pinto beans, black-eyed peas, and navy beans) and bean products (such as tofu) are rich in calcium and vegetable protein.

Seaweed contains high amounts of calcium, phosphorus, magnesium, boron, iron, iodine, and sodium. It also contains vitamins A, B1, C, E, and is one of the few vegetarian sources of vitamin B12. Calcium and magnesium content in common foods is listed in the table on the next page.

CALCIUM AND MAGNESIUM IN FOODS		
SOURCE	Calcium (mg)	Magnesium (mg)
Barley (1 cup, cooked)	17	35
Beet greens (1 cup, boiled)	164	98
Bok choy (1 cup)	158	19
Broccoli (1 cup, boiled)	72	37
Brown rice (1 cup, cooked)	20	84
Brussels sprouts (1 cup, cooked)	56	31
Butternut squash (1 cup, boiled)	46	22
Chickpeas (1 cup, cooked)	80	79
Collards (1 cup, boiled)	226	32
Dates, dried (1 cup)	57	62
Figs, dried (10 medium)	275	110
Green beans (1 cup, boiled)	58	31
Kale (1 cup, boiled)	94	23
Kidney beans (1 cup, boiled)	50	80
Lentils (1 cup, boiled)	38	71
Lima beans (1 cup, boiled)	32	81
Molasses, blackstrap (1 Tbsp.)	172	43
Mustard greens (1 cup, boiled)	104	21
Navel orange (1 medium)	52	13
Navy beans (1 cup, boiled)	127	107
Oatmeal, instant (1 packet)	163	42
Okra (1 cup, boiled)	101	91
Pinto beans (1 cup, boiled)	82	94
Rhubarb, frozen, cooked	348	29
Raisins (1 cup)	71	48
Soybeans (1 cup, boiled)	175	148
Tofu (1/4 block)	131	37
Turnip greens (1 cup, boiled)	197	32
Vegetarian baked beans (1 cup)	127	81
White beans (1 cup, boiled)	191	134

Source: *USDA Nutrient Database*

Vitamin K

Bone contains significant amounts of vitamin K, and low levels of vitamin K have been found in the blood of those with osteoporosis and in postmenopausal women. Vitamin K is required for the production of osteocalcin, a protein that attracts calcium to bone tissue and facilitates beneficial calcium crystal formation. Vitamin K supplements have been shown to increase this process (known as carboxylation) in postmenopausal women, thereby reducing bone loss. In controlled trials, people with low bone density given large amounts of vitamin K (45 milligrams per day) showed an increase in bone density after six months, and decreased bone loss after one year [44].

Studies link insufficient vitamin K intake to fracture. Research at Harvard University found that women who consumed less than 109 micrograms a day sustained 30 percent more hip fractures over a 10-year period [45]. In the Framingham Heart Study between 1988 and 1995, 888 elderly men and women consumed various levels of vitamin K. Those averaging 56 micrograms per day experienced more hip fractures by 1995 than those reporting the highest intake levels of 254 micrograms per day. Researchers observe that vitamin K activates at least three proteins involved in bone health [46].

Broccoli is a great source of vitamin K, as are leafy greens, legumes, and soybean oil. Scientists have known for years that astronauts lose bone density rapidly in space. A report in 2000 found a lack of vitamin K in astronauts, which may directly contribute to the space-related bone loss [47]. Because intestinal bacteria make 90 percent of vitamin K, people who have had frequent or long-term antibiotic use are likely to have insufficient vitamin K. Vitamin K is fat-soluble, and can be malabsorbed by those with chronic malabsorption or gastrointestinal problems.

Manganese

Manganese is a trace mineral, which is required for bone mineralization and the formation of connective tissue in cartilage and bone. In a study of Belgian women with osteoporosis (low BMD), blood levels of manganese were 75 percent lower than those of women without osteoporosis [48]. Manganese is toxic in high doses. The RDA is between 15 milligrams and 20 milligrams. Excellent sources of manganese include pecans, peanuts, pineapple fruit and juice, oatmeal, beans (pinto, lima, navy), rice, spinach, sweet potato, and whole wheat bread.

Zinc

Zinc, along with vitamin A and vitamin C, is essential for the formation of collagen. It enhances the biochemical action of vitamin D. Zinc levels have been found to be low in elderly people with osteoporosis. In one study, men consuming only 10 milligrams of zinc per day had almost twice the risk of osteoporotic fractures compared with those with significantly more zinc in their diets [49]. It has not yet been proven that zinc supplementation will prevent osteoporosis, but many doctors recommend that their patients supplement with 10-30 milligrams daily. Zinc is found in whole grain products, wheat bran and germ, brewer's yeast, and pumpkin seeds.

Copper
Copper is needed for normal bone synthesis and is a factor in the strengthening of connective bone tissue. A placebo-controlled two-year study reported that 3 milligrams of copper daily prevented bone loss [50]. Although more research is required to confirm the role of copper in treating osteoporosis, many nutritionists recommend two to three milligrams per day, especially if the person is supplementing with zinc, as zinc will deplete copper levels. Copper is found naturally in liver, shellfish, leafy vegetables, legumes, grains, and spirulina. Water that is delivered through copper piping is also a good source.

Strontium
Strontium, the trace mineral (not to be confused with the radioactive substance of the same name), plays a crucial role in bone remodeling. It tends to migrate to sites in bone where active remodeling is taking place. Several small studies have observed decreased bone pain, and an increase in bone formation in people taking quite high doses of strontium [51]. Most experts recommend between 1 and

3 milligrams per day. The drug Strontium Ranelate, appears to reduce the incidence of vertebral fractures in postmenopausal women with low bone density.

(See Chapter 6 for more information on Strontium Ranelate)

Boron

Boron, a trace element, appears to play an important role in bone building and strength. It has a role in parathyroid metabolism and influences the functions of calcium, magnesium, vitamin D, and phosphorus. Supplementation has been shown to increase the level of estrogen in some women. In a 1987 study, women taking 3 milligrams of supplemental boron for seven weeks lost 44 percent less calcium and 33 percent less magnesium in their urine than those not taking boron [52]. Boron deficiency has also been linked to arthritis, and there are indications that supplemental boron may provide relief. In areas where soil levels of boron are high, it has been noted that arthritis incidence is lower [53].

Boron is safe when taken at the recommended daily dosage of 2 to 6 milligrams. It is found in sea vegetables, leafy vegetables, avocados, legumes, and nuts. Wine has also been shown to contain appreciable amounts of boron.

Silicon

Silicon is important for skin, hair, and in the formation of connective tissue, bone, and cartilage. The trace mineral combines with calcium and is highly concentrated at sites of growing bones. In preliminary research, supplementation with silicon increased bone mineral density in a group of eight women with low bone density [54]. Silica is found in hard, unprocessed grains and vegetables, especially cabbage, parsnips, asparagus, olives, and radishes. Horsetail and oatstraw teas are excellent sources of silica.

Betain

Individuals with osteoporosis often absorb calcium poorly. Low stomach acid (hypochlorhydria) is relatively common in women over the age of 50, and may reduce absorption of most forms of calcium. Betain is an acidifying agent for the entire gastrointestinal system that increases the absorption of bone building nutrients. It is found in specific supplements.

Folic Acid, Vitamin B6, Vitamin B12
These three are known to reduce levels of the amino acid homocysteine in the body. Homocystinuria, a condition associated with high homocysteine levels, is known to cause osteoporosis. Although no research exists on the effects of supplementation, normal amounts found in high-potency B-complex supplements should be adequate [55]. Pyroxidine (vitamin B6) is required for collagen linking and the strength of connective bone tissue.

Foliate(the form of folic acid found in foods) can be added to the diet through green, leafy vegetables, beans, and citrus fruits. Whole grain cereals, green cruciferous vegetables, lean meats and chicken, and dairy foods are good sources of vitamin B6 and B12.

Vitamin A & Vitamin C
Your body uses these to make collagen, which keeps bones flexible and strong. Animal studies have shown that

osteoporosis can result from vitamin C deficiency [56].

Too much vitamin A, however, can be harmful. High serum levels of retinol (vitamin A) are associated with an increased risk for hip fracture in men, suggesting that the popularity of foods fortified with vitamin A may need to be reviewed [57]. Earlier studies suggest that vitamin A may prevent the formation of new bone and increase the risk of fractures. A Swedish study examined 247 women with hip fracture as compared with 873 women in a control group. Researchers found that, for every one milligram-per-day (3,333 IU) increase in vitamin A (retinol), the risk of hip fracture increased by 68 percent. While it is essential for the formation of collagen, excessive dietary intake of vitamin A appears to be linked to an increased risk for hip fracture [58]. Most fruits have high vitamin C content – especially citrus fruits, berries, apples, pineapples, and tomatoes.

Vitamin E

It is known that free radical activity may increase bone resorption. A preliminary report on the effectiveness of vitamin E in preventing bone loss in animals suggests that supplementation may be a way to reverse free-radical damage in bone [59]. Good sources of vitamin E include wheat germ, sunflower seeds, pine nuts, sun-dried tomatoes, and almonds.

Essential Fatty Acids

Supplementing with fish oil may improve calcium metabolism in older women with osteoporosis. A preliminary study examined older women of average age 80 with osteoporosis (low BMD) who took 4 grams of fish oil (gamma-linolenic acid) every day for four months. Researchers found that the women had higher blood levels of calcium, improved calcium absorption, and chemicals in their urine indicating bone formation. When fish oil was combined with evening primrose oil (gamma-linoleic acid), there was an increase in bone density of 3.1 percent over a three-year period [60]. This is a significant outcome in older women, and more research is needed in this important area.

Bone Care Nutrients

A well-balanced diet provides the best source of nutrients. If your diet is inadequate, or you wish to make sure you are getting the essentials, you might consider a mineral and vitamin supplement. Consult your health-care provider to help ascertain which supplement is best for you. Be aware that certain vitamin and mineral supplements can interact with medications.

Summary

Research indicates that dietary and lifestyle choices influence bone strength and health. A fundamental prevention and treatment strategy includes a diet that emphasizes the consumption of fresh vegetables, leafy greens, vegetable proteins, and avoids refined foods, heavy meats, caffeine, and carbonated drinks. The adequate intake of essential bone nutrients is also essential. These approaches will benefit overall health, as well as bone health. Indeed, embracing a healthy diet, receiving recommended amounts of vitamins and minerals, and adhering to a regular exercise program may be the most effective means to prevent bone loss and fragility fracture.

***

Chapter 11
A Family Story, 16 Years Later

Living with low bone density.

In three decades, osteoporosis has gone from being a rare bone disease to being a major health threat. The World Health Organization predicts a global epidemic of osteoporosis by 2050, and the National Osteoporosis Foundation warns of fragility fractures occurring every 20 seconds in the United States. A proliferation of glossy advertisements and celebrity endorsements encourages fearful mid-life women to adopt bone density screening and bone-sparing drugs to avert debilitating hip fracture and painful curvature of the spine. The message has been so compelling it is not surprising that physicians and their patients have universally accepted it.

While medicine, at its core, is about preventing and healing illness, medicine is also about big business — billions of dollars annually. Giant public relations machines promote treatments and cures, but they increasingly promote diseases and epidemics as well. Marketing campaigns often capitalize on people's fears of aging and illness. Osteoporosis exemplifies this. It has become one of the most commercially profitable diseases ever because it diagnoses and treats the well. Healthy women and men throughout the world have been convinced that by virtue of normal, age-related bone loss, they are at risk for a serious disease.

It simply isn't true.

Here are the facts:

* Loss of bone density is a normal aspect of growing older and is a condition that may never manifest as disease.

* Most people who have low bone density will not fracture, and the majority of fractures occur in people who do not have osteoporosis (low BMD).

* Hip fractures — the real fear surrounding osteoporosis — result from many contributing factors. Preventing falls in the elderly will decrease hip fractures far more effectively than drugs to treat low bone density.

* Most osteoporosis drugs do not help the majority of people taking them and in some cases may exacerbate a patient's

condition. They can carry risks that may surface years later

* The best bone-strengthening treatments come from lifestyle choices each individual has control over: eating nutritious foods, getting regular exercise, lowering exposure to chemical toxins, and managing stress.

Modern medicine is an essential part of our lives. The vast majority of medical practitioners are compassionate caregivers who act sincerely in the best interests of their patients, and many people suffering acute and serious diseases benefit greatly from medical intervention. However, medical intervention, specifically drug treatment, must be administered on the basis of sound research and study – and with careful assessment of the benefits and risks. The risks cannot be understated. Prescription drugs cause more than 106,000 deaths annually in the United States.

Physicians bear a tremendous responsibility in administering care, and patients bear an equally large responsibility – their own health. We must cultivate a healthy, open-minded skepticism and willingness to question diagnoses, while educating ourselves about the safety and effectiveness of any treatment before embarking on it. By challenging and questioning current practices, we can contribute to creating greater rigor in science and better health care for all.

Living with Low Bone Density

There is no doubt that osteoporosis, characterized by fragility fractures, is a disease with potentially serious consequences. Established osteoporosis, however, is a rare disease linked to many factors. Osteoporosis, defined by low bone density alone, is a condition that most of us can live with and suffer no ill effects.

Eleven members of my family spanning three generations have a diagnosis of either osteoporosis or osteopenia. It is around 16 years since we were diagnosed, and although it is clear there is a genetic factor involved, there is still virtually nothing known about our condition. It is labeled "idiopathic" — of unknown cause. In this sense it differs from age-related osteoporosis as discussed in this book. It is interesting to observe however, that in all this time, few of us have fractured and the diagnosis has not limited our ability to enjoy life in any way.

My daughter was only 16 when she was told that she had the bones of an 80-year-old. In typical teenage style, she didn't discuss it much. Her father and I had little information on the disease and were very worried. She appeared to be getting on with her life, but years later told me that the diagnosis had affected her tremendously. She feared more painful fractures and cut back on physical activity, believing her fragile bones could not withstand any knocks or pressure. She avoided sports at school and no longer went skiing. She even gave up dancing, which was especially hard, as she had been passionate about it from an early age. All of this was quite the opposite of what she ought to have done — but no such advice was given.

As time went by and she continued to be fracture-free, my daughter's confidence returned. At 18, she graduated from high school in New Zealand and set off on a working holiday, backpacking through Asia and Europe working in London and travelling through India, and Nepal. She is now married and living in London and has a successful fashion photography business. She has had no fractures for 16 years.

My parents are fit and active, and both enjoy very good health. Their story has been told in a previous chapter. My brother has "severe" osteopenia. He farms a large block of land, and his lifestyle demands constant physical activity. He is extremely fit and enjoys competition tennis, badminton, skiing, and surfboarding. In 1988, he suffered multiple broken bones when his tractor rolled on him. He is lucky to have survived. These high-impact fractures, obviously, cannot be linked to osteoporosis. Testament to his good health, he made a complete recovery and remains fracture-free today. He tells me that he doesn't give a thought to his diagnosis of low bone density.

My son has very low bone density, enough to qualify him for a diagnosis of osteoporosis. Although he fractured his wrist in a heavy fall from gymnastics equipment at age 14 and twice broke a finger while playing basketball, he has remained fracture-free for 15 years. He lives with his family in Canada and has continued to be very active. He maintains that the diagnosis has not affected his life in any way.

My husband has bone density considerably lower than the threshold for osteoporosis, putting him in an "extreme risk" category. Yet, other than a minor crack in a wrist bone as a child, he has never fractured. He was very athletic when young, playing competition rugby and winning high-jump awards. He is a strong, healthy, physically active person who doesn't fit the image of a fragile person. He is a home handyman who balks at nothing — lifting heavy objects, climbing high trees to prune them, painting the roof, building fences, sheds, and furniture, gardening, and laying concrete and wooden floors. Interestingly, until I reminded him of his diagnosis, he had forgotten how supposedly serious it was. He was momentarily alarmed before shrugging his shoulders and dismissing it. He figures that by continuing to take care of his physical, mental, and spiritual health, he is doing the best that he can to avert future problems. Because so much is not known about osteoporosis, chances are that his bones are strong and flexible, and the low BMD reading is meaningless.

My last DXA scan (in 1996) indicated that I had "serious osteopenia," meaning low bone density, but not in the osteoporosis category. I had four non-serious wrist fractures as a child, and a wrist fracture in 2006 from which I have fully recovered.

I come from a family of gardeners. Gardening is great weight-bearing exercise that enhances flexibility and improves muscle and bone strength. My grandfather who lost a leg in the World War I was still digging his prolific garden when he was 90. My sister and her husband have a two-and-a-half-acre garden that they have single-handedly established over 35 years. They have woodlands, weeping pear trees, delicate maples, and primulasgrown from seed collected in China. There are massive oaks, established borders, native trees and grasses, and rare, exquisite alpine blooms. They have a huge vegetable garden and produce abundant organic vegetables and fruit year-round. They are adventurers too, and in recent years they have traveled the Karakoram Highway through the Hindu Kush Mountains from China to Pakistan; climbed the lower reaches of the Tibetan plateau on a botanical pilgrimage; survived high altitudes traveling in Tibet; and taken a boat down the mighty Mekong river in Laos, negotiating its waterways and canals where it reaches the ocean in Vietnam. Julie has osteopenia too, but she has never fractured. She is now in her early 60s and is very fit.

My oldest sister, now in her 60s has osteoporosis. She has been advised that she is at high risk of fracture and must take long-term bisphosphonate treatment. She is now grandmother to five granddaughters. She works part-time and is very involved with the community and her family. She and her husband have a beautiful, rural property and work their garden, growing trees, organic vegetables, and fruit, and beekeeping. She eats well, making sure that her diet includes lots of fresh vegetables, nuts, seeds, grains, and essential fatty acids. She has not had a fracture since she was 7 years old.

I do not dismiss the potential for problems for my son, daughter, and other family members later in life. Our history of childhood fracture and the very low bone density in some of us could increase our risk for fragility fracture. A dire prognosis, however, is far from confirmed: A wide biological variation in bone density exists among healthy adults; perhaps our low bone density is normal for us, and our bone strength and micro-architecture is sound. As medical science continues to grapple with understanding bone health over the course of a person's lifetime, no one can say what the future holds.

In setting out to learn all I could about osteoporosis I have uncovered myth and misinformation every step of the way. Thankfully, the status quo can change

There is now healthy debate in the medical community over the appropriateness of testing and treating well women for a disease that they may never have; and there are ongoing questions about the accuracy of diagnosis and about the safety and effectiveness of treatments.

My research has confirmed that we must each take responsibility for our well-beingand for making wise choices. I believe this book to be optimistic and reassuring. I hope that it gives women the courage to deeply question their physicians, and that it encourages them to continue on their own journey of education and self-discovery. Menopause is not a disease; neither is growing old. These are rewarding years when we can take positive action to assure long and healthy lives.

***

CPSIA information can be obtained
at www.ICGtesting.com
Printed in the USA
BVHW051330180423
662564BV00013B/894